# YOGALOSOPHY

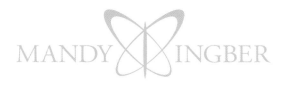

MANDY INGBER

# YOGALOSOPHY

## 28 Days to the Ultimate MIND-BODY MAKEOVER

SEAL PRESS

Yogalosophy
28 Days to the Ultimate Mind-Body Makeover

Published by Seal Press
A Member of the Perseus Books Group
1700 Fourth Street
Berkeley, CA 94710

Library of Congress Cataloging-in-Publication Data

Ingber, Mandy.
   Yogalosophy : 28 days to the ultimate mind-body makeover / by Mandy
Ingber.
      pages cm
   ISBN 978-1-58005-445-4
1.  Yoga--Philosophy. 2.  Physical fitness. 3.  Mind and body. 4.
Motion
picture actors and actresses--Health and hygiene--United States.  I.
Title.
   RA781.67.I54 2013
   613.7'1--dc23
                              2012038589


10  9  8  7  6  5  4  3  2

Cover design by Erin Seaward-Hiatt
Interior design by Megan Cooney and Tabitha Lahr
Photographs of Mandy Ingber by Javiera Estrada Photography
Location: Kinevision Studio in Venice, California
Printed in the United States of America
Distributed by Publishers Group West

*"Out beyond ideas of wrongdoing and rightdoing, there is a field. I'll meet you there."*

—RUMI

*This book is dedicated to my father.*

# CONTENTS

# PART 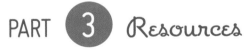 3 Resources

"Having the body you want begins with loving the body you have."

— MANDY INGBER

# INTRODUCTION

## YOGALOSOPHY:
### 28 Days to the Ultimate Mind-body Makeover

**W**hat if I told you that you already have the perfect body?

Okay, stop rolling your eyes. I know, I know. It's hard to believe this at first, but don't close the book yet. Humor me for a moment. Just by opening this book, you have initiated the process of change.

You might have heard of Yogalosophy through magazines because of the A-list actors with healthy, fit bodies, like Jennifer Aniston and Kate Beckinsale, who use it and get results. Maybe you picked up this book because Jennifer Aniston looks so fresh and healthy, so comfortable in her own skin that you're thinking, *I'll have what she's having*. But what if the body you want is already in the room with you? It may just be hiding under a layer or two. This sounds radical, and it is, but when you begin to focus on your best body, which is already strong, healthy, and in shape, your body responds.

I ought to know—I have been all over the map with my relationship to my body. I have had times in my life when I've been extremely thin, then overweight; when I have been injured and unable to perform my normal exercise routine; and times when I have worked out for hours on end. All of this has taught me that the body is a work in progress. Since I designed and began following this course in positive reinforcement, which I call Yogalosophy, fifteen years ago, I have never had a major weight fluctuation.

But conceptualizing and practicing Yogalosophy didn't come easily. Before that, there was a period of time when I went through a lot of stressful stuff all at once. I'd been injured, and then, on top of that, I was physically assaulted by random attackers and was beaten so severely I required two surgeries. The pain and trauma were a lot to handle. I had already used food as a way to cope in the past, so I ate unconsciously and gained an excessive amount of weight—I'm talking fifty pounds, which on a five-foot-four frame qualifies as a lot. I didn't want to deal with anybody or anything. As a signal to the rest of the world to "stay away," I started wearing pajamas wherever I went. Even footy pajamas. I kid you not. Yes. Instead of clothes. Even on a trip through Europe, it was in PJs.

One night, after the Italy section of my European feeding frenzy, I hit a point where I realized I felt extremely heavy and uncomfortable in my skin. It was then that the thought came to me that I was ready to lose weight—I'd hit my limit; I was no longer able to sustain this level of discomfort. Since the weight gain, I'd avoided looking at myself, so I took off the pajamas I had worn to dinner and stood naked, eyes closed, in front of the mirror. I took a deep breath, opened my eyes, and looked at myself for the first time in a long time. Only, I did not cast a judgmental glare upon myself. I looked with love and acceptance. Yes, there were folds of skin in places that had never been touching before, more chub around my arms and on my belly and all over my body, but it hit me that I still had the body I desired; it was just hiding underneath a couple of layers.

I kept that vision and began to focus on the perfect body that was already in the room with me . . . just hiding. And I began to talk positively to myself, instead of ignoring or beating myself up. That's how I started to break the pattern of self-sabotage that caused me to gain almost forty percent of my body mass: The voice that used to tell me "it's not good enough" or "it used to be better" was replaced with a coach that would breathe and take it one encouraging moment at a time. Choosing what a healthy, thin person would choose, instead of giving up as I had.

Ultimately, I took my lessons and began teaching them to others, including those celebrities with the enviable bodies. Everything I learned and continue to teach them is in this book. I designed *Yogalosophy: 28 Days to the Ultimate Mind-body Makeover* as an action plan to repattern your habits, to develop new, positive self-talk, and help you to channel your emotions. You'll see that I also refer to this handbook, this way of life, as the Y28 Revolution. You'll find here all the stuff that's helped me—and my students—achieve healthy, fit bodies and fulfilling (self-loving) lives. This Y28 Revolution started with my body, but it is the same formula that has allowed me to accomplish my dreams.

Yogalosophy is more than just yoga, because yoga is only one of its modalities. In this program, you'll be using many different activities combined with yoga postures to tone your body and to feel better in general. I give you options, because if you're like me, no one thing feels right all the time. There are so many incredible ways to get into shape, and I've tried most of them. I coined the term Yogalosophy as a way to explain how I fuse it all together. Think of it as an attitude about uniting all the parts of yourself, a life approach inspired by the word *yoga,* which means "union" and *losophy* which means "knowledge." Yogalosophers bring the yoga practice of mindfulness and intention-setting into whatever they do. In this program, you only have to do one thing that is really, really hard. If you can do this one thing, you will be able to have what you want:

*Accept your body as already perfect.*

Don't believe it yet? I know. It's the most challenging thing in the book. I still go through times when I resist the idea of accepting myself the way I am, because I'm afraid if I accept something it will stay that way forever. The old thought process wants me to believe that if I accept myself, I won't be motivated to make change. What I've found is that when I really accept things as they are, I have choices. The truth is, nothing ever stays the same. Everything changes over time, right? Now, I understand I have a part in the direction I want change to go.

As an instructor, I've given health and fitness advice to women with some of the most admired bodies in Hollywood, and I'm telling you honestly that you are no different than they are. You have the exact same four components as your favorite stars. Here they are:

1 BODY: a physical body that needs to be cared for

2 WILLPOWER: a mind as a compass

3 EMOTIONS: feelings that will motivate you

4 ME!

And now I come in a handbook you can refer to again and again. How convenient is that?

I created *Yogalosophy: 28 Days to the Ultimate Mind-body Makeover* as a practical plan for starting fresh, no matter what your level of fitness may be. It's a twenty-eight-day revolution; the Y28 Revolution. They say it takes twenty-eight days to break a habit. I find that it's long enough to reset yourself but short enough so that you reach your goals and stay motivated.

For the next four weeks, you'll follow the Y28 Revolution routine, which includes guidelines for eating lean, healthy food. You get options so you can handle it. You also have optional add-ons to the basic Yogalosophy workout, and the three diet options can be integrated into the program or not, depending on wherever you are in your life right now. This will help you toward your goals and motivate you to keep going because, let's be real, our needs and moods tend to be cyclical. Some days I have a lot of energy, while other days I want nothing more than to curl up, eat a bag of potato chips, and Facebook stalk! Every day, though, I can consciously act in a way that moves me toward my goals. In a spiral!

On top of that, this program brings together new insights, additional exercises, yoga pose variations, and life lessons particular to each of the twenty-eight days. These twenty-eight instructions will help you revolutionize the way you approach your fitness and health, and keep you on the journey back to yourself.

So, wow, we've got a lot to do. Let's get started. . . . Take the risk, turn the page . . . Let's go!

PART 1

# Practical Guidelines

# HOW TO USE THIS BOOK

You don't need anyone to tell you that when you work out more and eat the right foods in moderation you will lose weight and tone up. You know that already, right? Since my moods go in cycles, and I am not motivated by the same things every day, I use a balance between a consistent workout routine and variation in approach. Doing the same thing in the same way every day will not yield the best results, because you are different each day. That is the beauty of this program. Each day offers an opportunity to approach wellness in a new way, and is structured to provide both consistency and change.

Everyone has their own personal rhythm, a time of day when we get sleepy or feel energized, get hungry or even feel lonely. You aren't expected to be entirely positive and ready to work out every day. It's important to notice and embrace your shifting feelings rather than write them off or ignore them. They are your secret weapons, and this book will help you leverage them to generate the energy required to see changes in your body.

They say it takes twenty-eight days to break or create a habit. In general, there is a twenty-eight-day (or so) lunar cycle that affects the ebb and flow of the tides of the ocean, farmers' crops, and women's menstrual cycles. The emotional biorhythms, our emotional arcs, work in twenty-eight-day cycles too, which is why I have designed this program for twenty-eight days.

So how does it work? There are three components to the program: 1. the Yogalosophy Routine; 2. the Diet Plan; and 3. the Daily Activities. Every day is shaped by a unique lesson, or "intention," for the heart, mind, body, and spirit, which informs the routine and the activities. Start each day by reading the lesson, and then follow the activities in the Action Checklist.

This is the core of the program, and it includes the Yogalosophy routine and a directive about how to use the day's intention to guide you through your activities. In addition to the Action Checklist, each day includes bonus poses, an extra credit activity, a daily recipe, and optional activities that reinforce the day's theme. These include keeping a daily journal and writing a daily gratitude list, which supports the physical work through self-knowledge. These extra activities don't start all at once! As you ease into the program, I will introduce them one at a time, giving you time to incorporate the fundamentals of the Y28 Revolution into your daily life. Before you begin, select one of the optional meal plans from the back of the book. Be sure to choose one you feel comfortable maintaining for the twenty-eight-day cycle.

Read the following sections for more details about each component of the program and how to apply them each day.

## ACTION CHECKLIST

This is where it all begins! This is where you tune-in to the daily intention and get your mind and body moving. It's the core of the program each day, with a touch of musical fun to round it out:

INTENTION: This is the lens through which you approach your routine. Each day's intention reflects the day's theme, or focus. Applying the intention helps you leverage your emotions to fuel your workout.

PLAYLIST: Each day, I provide a sample playlist of music that sets the tone for the daily intention. The playlists are optional! You don't necessarily have to download each song. Feel free to create your own playlists.

YOGALOSOPHY ROUTINE VARIATION: On most days, I'll offer optional variations to the standard Yogalosophy routine of poses and toners. I recommend that you follow these variations whenever possible, since they not only build on strength work you've done on preceding days, but they also reflect and reinforce the intention of the day.

CARDIO OPTION: Getting your heart rate up is important to overall health and body maintenance, and it also lifts the spirit. The cardio workouts range from a brisk walk or hike, to running or taking a spin class. To maximize the benefits of the program, it's important to incorporate cardio into your daily routine. This will also shift your attitude by clearing out any emotional debris.

# EXTRA ACTIVITIES

Your body is not simply made of the foods that you eat or solely shaped by the exercise you do. Your brain chemistry and emotions have much more power over the desired result than you may realize. The following activities and exercises are optional, but they are the magic of the program, the "losophy." They support the physical work you do. As you do these exercises and get to know yourself, you will work from a wisdom that is unique to you. Feel free to take what you like and set the rest aside. Trust your process.

POSE(S) OF THE DAY: In addition to the Yogalosophy Routine and cardio, I will provide a daily bonus pose—or several—to incorporate into that day's workout regimen. In some cases, they will serve as that day's variation to the Yogalosophy Routine.

EXTRA CREDIT: These are fun and rewarding activities that reflect the day's intention. The purpose is not only to reintroduce the theme of the day, but also to reward your daily efforts.

JOURNALING: This optional activity provides an opportunity for self-reflection and reinforces the theme of the day. On some days, I'll provide a writing prompt. Otherwise, let the Daily Intention be your guide. Spend at least ten minutes writing each day.

GRATITUDE LIST: We have so much to be grateful for! This activity helps foster self-esteem and a deeper awareness of our blessings. Make a list of at least five things you're grateful for each day. Some days, I'll provide prompts. Otherwise, focus on what you're grateful for about YOU. Let the Daily Intention be your guide.

BREATHING EXERCISES: On Day 6, I introduce a series of breathing exercises that are intended to ground and center you, and connect you with your life-force energy, not only during your workouts but also any time you need to find balance or calm in your day. I recommend incorporating them at the beginning or end of your daily Yogalosophy Routine.

Now that you have the lay of the land, you are ready for the Y28 Revolution! Just remember, be loving and gentle with yourself. There is nothing set in stone. Your body is a beautiful work in progress.

# YOGALOSOPHY ROUTINE

**A**s you go through this program, you will find special exercises or poses to try on each day. However, the foundation for your exercise starts with a basic routine, shown on the following pages. Unless otherwise noted, you should start with this practice before moving on to the pose(s) of the day. As promised, I've offered variations to the daily routine, so you can mix it up a bit as you go through the Y28 Revolution.

I developed Yogalosophy, my signature hybrid-yoga routine, as the answer to a call. Yoga can be very intimidating, even for me. My father could wrap both legs around his head; he could also meditate standing up for ninety minutes, twice a day. I am a different animal. I want to know that what I do is enough, without having to prove something by performing party tricks or setting lofty goals for myself. In short, I have found that the more consistent and moderate I am, the less my body fluctuates and the more effortlessly I seem to find balance. I have accessed the powerful healing and strengthening benefits of yoga and paired them with complementary toners, which engage the smaller, less-used muscle groups, to help you get into the best shape in the minimal amount of time. Add a dash of cardio, and the outcome is maximum benefits with minimal effort!

Each component of the program gives action to part of a growth cycle. You will use your mental, emotional, and physical self. You might not feel amazing every single day. Good! Show up to the best of your ability and start over again the next day. You will see. Exercise, wellness, and fitness form a cumulative process. You may hit a plateau for several days, and then suddenly, BREAKTHROUGH.

## THE YOGALOSOPHY WORKOUT

This routine can accommodate any level of fitness, so don't worry if you're not already a yogini or have never taken a yoga class! Just take your time, breathe, and make sure you are aligned properly. It takes time to gain strength. The more you practice, the more comfortable you will be in the positions. Soon, you'll see your stamina increase. So go easy and start with one set of each posture. Hold each pose for thirty to sixty seconds or six to eight deep breaths.

Follow this with a set of the Yogalosophy toners. Each toner should be done for eight repetitions followed by eight pulsing reps. Build up to two sets of each. Part of this practice includes listening to and respecting your body, so feel free to add or reduce the work according to how you feel.

## MOUNTAIN POSE/CALF RAISES

Begin with legs and feet together. Spread your toes and cover as much ground as you can with your feet. Roll your shoulders back and down, turning the palms open as you naturally allow the shoulders to externally rotate. Lengthen your spine by drawing the navel in, and extend your chest toward the sky as you gently drop your tailbone to aim toward your heels. Breathe. Hold for six to eight breaths.

When you feel ready, bring your hands to your hips and press the balls of your feet into the floor, to lift your heels. This will engage and work the calves. When you press through the feet, keep your body nice and straight. Firm your legs. At the end of eight reps, keep your heels lifted and pulse up for eight reps. This works the abdominals and calves, and centers you.

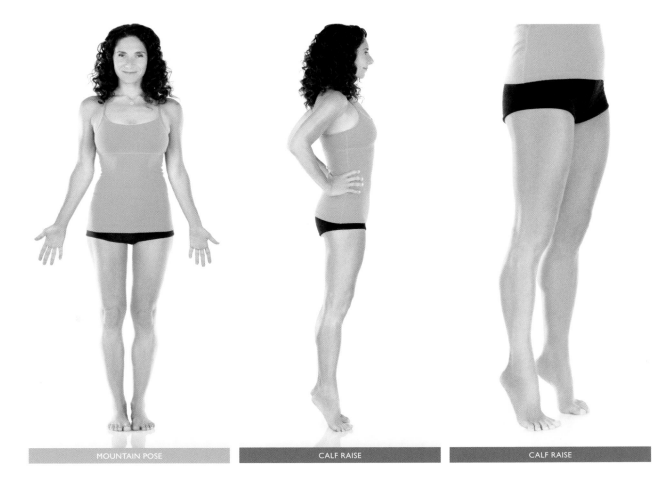

MOUNTAIN POSE          CALF RAISE          CALF RAISE

## CHAIR/SQUATS

Either keep the feet together or separate hip-width apart. Extend your arms by your ears, palms facing inward. As you lower your hips down into an imaginary chair, shift your weight back so that when you look down, you can still see your toes. Lift your chest so that you peel your belly off of your thighs. Hold and take eight deep breaths.

Bring your hands by your hips, or wherever feels comfortable. Separate the feet wider than hip-width. Lower your butt back and down and then squeeze your glutes and inner thighs to lift up. These are squats. Make sure that the feet are parallel, with toes pointing straight ahead. When you shift back into the squat, keep the knees aligned over the center of the feet. At the end of eight reps, make the movement smaller (about three inches) and pulse for eight.

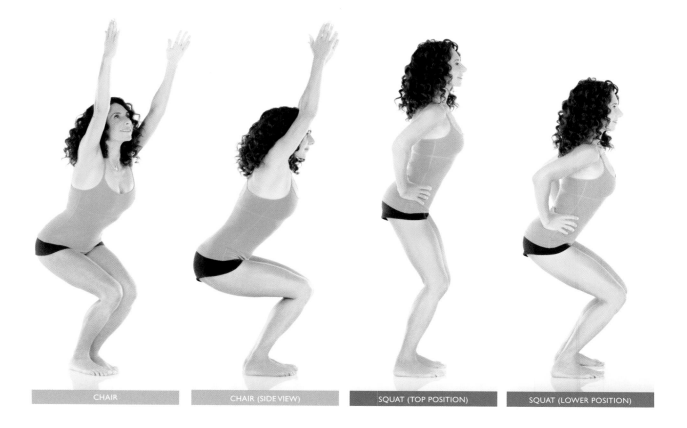

CHAIR     CHAIR (SIDE VIEW)     SQUAT (TOP POSITION)     SQUAT (LOWER POSITION)

## CRESCENT/LUNGES

Step your left leg back three to five feet (or as far back as it can comfortably go), keeping the feet hip-width apart for balance, as if you are on a railroad track instead of a tightrope. Bend your right (front) leg to a ninety-degree angle, with the knee tracking directly over the center of the foot and the back (left) heel lifted off of the floor. Square your hips forward and sweep your arms up overhead with palms facing each other. Think back to Mountain pose and remember to elongate your spine as you gently drop the tailbone down. Soften the ribcage in toward your spine and reach out through your sternum as you find extension. Relax the shoulders down away from the ears. Feel the two opposing forces of gravity and extension working to hold you in alignment. Breathe eight breaths.

Step your back foot forward a few inches and bend your back knee. Bring your hands to your hips and lower your back knee toward the floor. After you lunge for eight reps, make the movement smaller and pulse for eight. (After you repeat the Crescent/Lunge combo two times, step the back leg up to meet the front leg and switch to side two.)

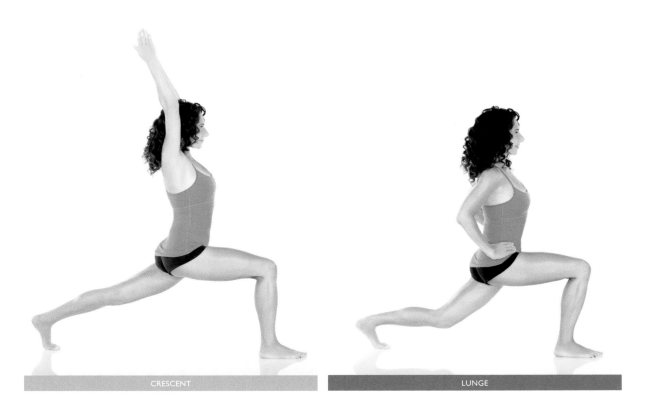

CRESCENT

LUNGE

## TEMPLE/PLIÉ SQUATS

Step your feet wide apart. Angle your toes out so that they are at the ten o'clock and two o'clock positions. Lower your tush down as if you are sitting onto a bench. Keep your torso upright with head, shoulders, hips, knees, and feet on one line. Lower down as much as you can so that the tush is as low as the knees. (Don't worry if you can't go that low; it's just a guideline). Press your knees open, making sure your knees are not buckling in but turned outward. You should feel this engage the glutes. Press your palms together in front of the heart in a prayer position. Lean the torso back to maintain the extension out through the crown of the head. Hold for eight breaths.

Bring your hands to your hips and press to standing. Then lower down with control until your hips are at knee level. Repeat eight times, then pulse the plié squat for eight reps. Bonus move: At the end of the reps, hold the squat and press the knees out and open, engaging the outer glutes. Repeat.

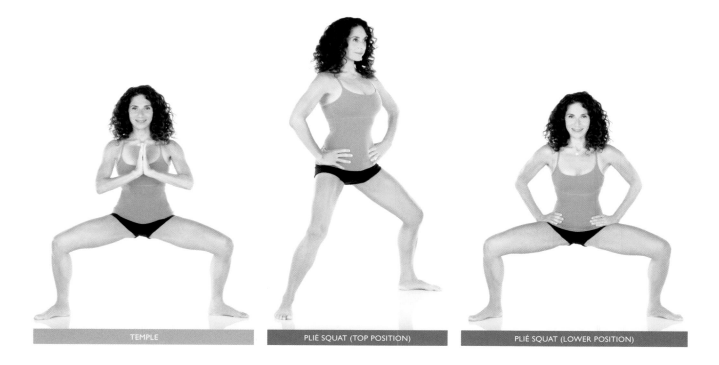

TEMPLE · PLIÉ SQUAT (TOP POSITION) · PLIÉ SQUAT (LOWER POSITION)

## DOWNWARD FACING DOG/EXTENDED LEG LIFTS

Step your feet together at the top of your mat. Fold yourself forward, and place your hands on the mat, shoulder-width apart. Walk your legs back behind you and aim your hips up at a diagonal so that you are in an inverted "V" shape. Press through your palms and the heels of your hands. Lift your sit bones up to the ceiling as you press your chest toward your thighs, allowing the shoulders to open and the heels to sink toward the mat. Make sure your spine is straight. If you need to bend your knees or raise your heels in order to do so, that is okay. Hold for eight breaths.

From Downward Facing Dog, extend your leg into a high leg lift behind you and point your right toes, angling them slightly out to the right as you raise your leg. Slowly lift and lower, tapping the toe on the floor as you lower. Engage the muscles where the back of your thigh and your butt meet. At the end of eight reps, pulse it for eight and repeat. Move back to Downward Facing Dog. Take eight breaths and switch sides.

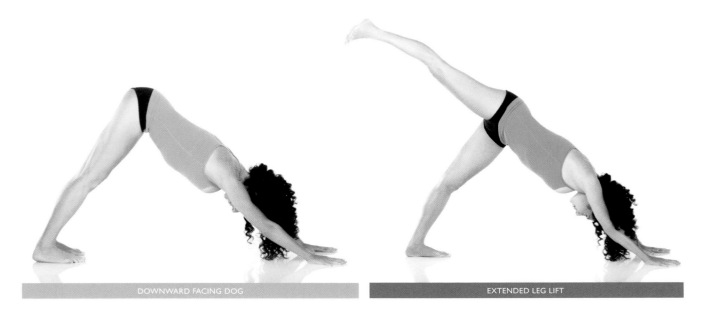

DOWNWARD FACING DOG

EXTENDED LEG LIFT

## CAT COW/SIDE LEG-LIFTS

Lower your knees to the floor so that you are on your hands and knees in a tabletop position. Place your palms directly below your shoulders, with knees directly below your hips. Maintain a neutral spine for a couple of breaths. Soften your ribs toward your spine (you can do this by exhaling sharply; feel the breath draw the ribs in) and find the natural extension from your spine, out through the top of your head. On the inhale, arch your back. Roll your shoulders back and down to engage the lateral muscles that run down the side of the body as you lift your chin up, and at the same time, lift the sit bones up. This is an expansion of the lungs, rib cage, and chest. On the exhale, push your palms into the floor and tilt your tailbone under, making your torso concave. Lower your chin to your chest and lift the naval toward your spine. Inhale while arching, and exhale while contracting, like a Halloween cat.

Once you have done four reps of each, place your forearms on the mat. Tuck your pelvis down. Place your right hand out to the right side for support. Keep your legs bent at a ninety-degree angle, and raise your right leg straight out to the side. Lower the right knee to meet the left knee. Repeat eight times. Then pulse for eight. Do two sets. Repeat Cat/Cow and switch sides.

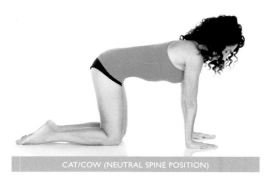

CAT/COW (NEUTRAL SPINE POSITION)

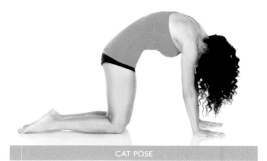

CAT POSE

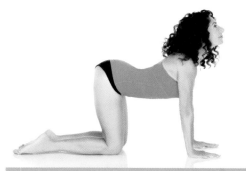

COW POSE

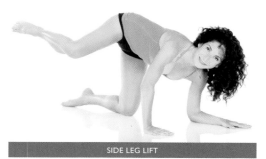

SIDE LEG LIFT

## BOW/SUPERMAN

Lie flat on your belly. Reach behind your back and interlace your fingers as you clasp your hands. Tuck your tailbone down slightly and bring your legs together. Inhale, and lift as much of your body off of the mat as you can. Exhale as you bring the hands down by the hips. Hold the pose for eight breaths. If you feel you are flexible enough, bend your knees and reach back for the tops of your feet or ankles. On an inhale, raise your thighs and chest high up off of the mat, pressing your feet into your hands to open the shoulders. Hold for eight breaths. Lower down.

Extend your arms out to the sides. At the same time, inhale and raise your torso up, feeling the muscles in your back engage. Continue to draw the shoulders away from the ears as you work here. Lift and lower eight times. Pulse for eight at the height of your range, then repeat.

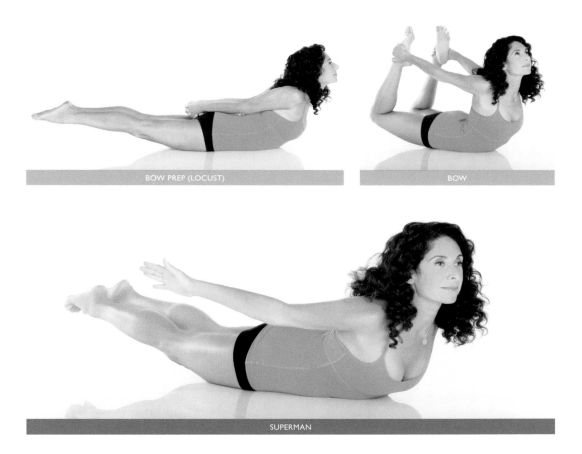

BOW PREP (LOCUST)

BOW

SUPERMAN

## OPTIONAL CORE STRENGTH

Slide your hands alongside your body so that your thumbs are directly below the chest. Hug your elbows in and shrug your shoulders back. Tuck the toes under and flex your thighs. On the exhale, push yourself off of the mat to a low plank by raising your entire torso up so that the elbows and shoulders are in alignment. Press up to a full push-up, or Plank position.

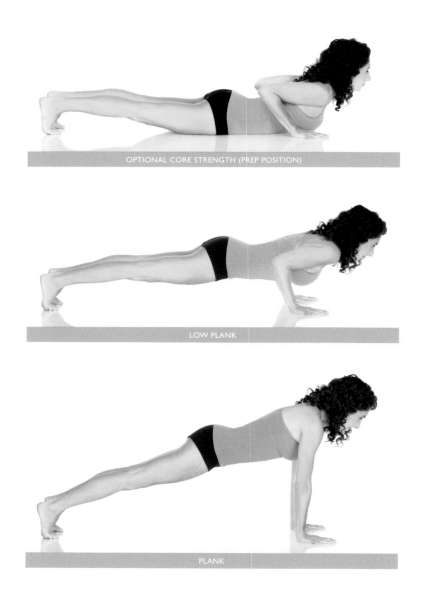

OPTIONAL CORE STRENGTH (PREP POSITION)

LOW PLANK

PLANK

## PLANK/PUSH-UPS

With your weight balanced equally between both palms and balls of the feet, flex your thighs and draw the navel in. Imagine that you are in Mountain Pose, so extend out through your sternum, soften the ribcage toward your spine, and send the tailbone down toward your heels. Look straight ahead about two feet.

After eight breaths, either bring your knees to the floor, keeping your abs engaged, or stay in Plank, hugging the elbows toward the side of your body as you lower your body down. Press back up without locking the elbows so that you keep the work in the muscles. Repeat the push-up eight times, and then pulse for eight. Repeat the entire set.

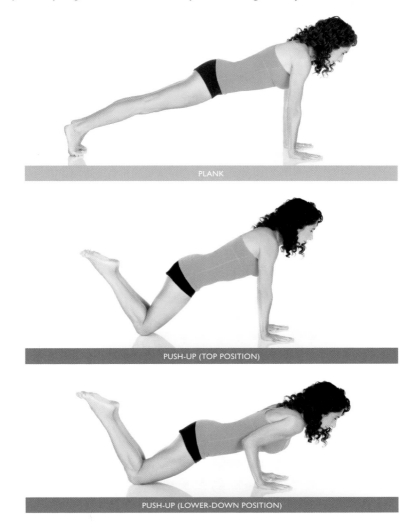

PLANK

PUSH-UP (TOP POSITION)

PUSH-UP (LOWER-DOWN POSITION)

## SIDE PLANK/TRICEP PUSH-UPS

From Plank, walk your right palm directly below your face and balance onto the right palm at the same time as you stack your feet and rock onto the outside of the right foot. Press your palm into the mat and press your hips up, which will lift the underside of your waist. Extend your left arm straight up, palm facing forward, so that it is in line with your right arm. Find the Mountain Pose in your Side Plank by scooping the tailbone, sending the sit bones to the heels. Align the head, shoulder, hips, and heels as you look up to the top hand. Switch sides. Hold for eight breaths on each side and repeat.

From your second set of Side Plank on the left side, bring your right hand behind you, so that the front of your body is now aiming toward the ceiling. Place the soles of the feet on the floor, and aim your fingers toward your heels so your elbows are facing behind you and you are in a tabletop position. From here, keep your elbows hugged in and lower down a few inches. Do eight reps of Tricep Push-ups and then eight pulses. Repeat twice. Lower your hips to the floor and lie down on your back.

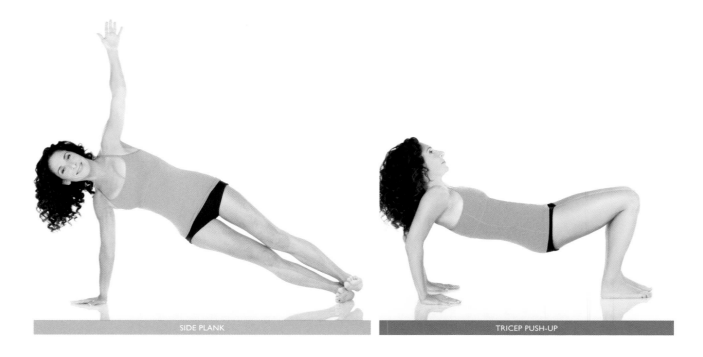

SIDE PLANK                    TRICEP PUSH-UP

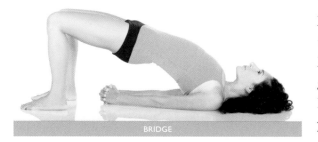

BRIDGE

## BRIDGE/PELVIC TUCKS

Lie on your back with feet parallel on the floor, hip-width apart. Slide your heels toward your tush so that you can graze your heels with your fingertips. Press your feet into the mat and peel your spine off the floor one vertebrae at a time. Press the hips up. Interlace your fingers underneath you as you wriggle onto your shoulders. Open up the front of your body and take eight breaths before you unclasp the hands and lower your hips to the floor.

Next, move into a Pelvic Tuck. Lower your hips to the floor and then squeeze your glutes as you press up full range of motion. After eight reps, squeeze in a tiny pulse at the top. Repeat two sets.

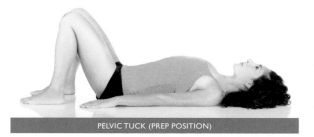

PELVIC TUCK (PREP POSITION)

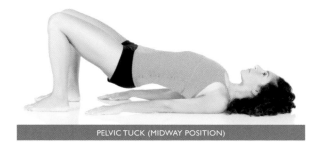

PELVIC TUCK (MIDWAY POSITION)

PELVIC TUCK (TOP POSITION)

## TWIST/CRISSCROSS ABS

Hug your right knee into your chest with both hands and then place your left palm on the outside of the right knee. Extend your right arm out to the side, palm facing down in the same line as the shoulder. Keep your right shoulder down on the floor and twist from your waist. Allow the knee to drop over to the left as you look over to your right hand. Breathe eight times and switch.

After you have repeated, bend both knees in to your chest and cross your ankles. Bring your hands behind your head and lift your head and your chest, drawing your right elbow to the outside of your left knee and then switch, drawing your left elbow to the outside of your right knee and crisscross with twisting abdominals, alternating sixteen on each side.

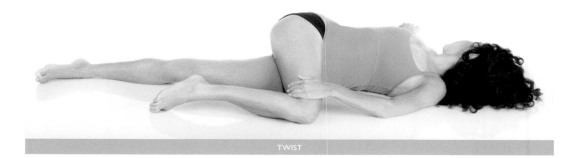

TWIST

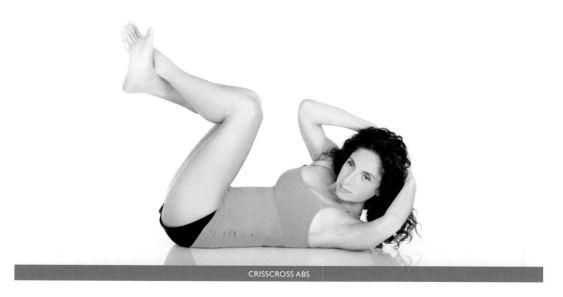

CRISSCROSS ABS

## BOAT/V-UPS

Sit up with the soles of your feet flat on the floor. Hook your hands behind your hamstrings and lean back slowly until you are balancing up on your sit bones. Lift your feet off of the ground and, with bent knees, bring your feet in alignment with your knees. Press your lower back in and extend your chest up to the sky. Release your hands from behind your hamstrings and reach your arms out in front of you, palms facing each other. Make sure you keep pressing your shoulders down. Breathe.

After eight breaths, lower both your upper body and your legs until they are hovering six inches above the mat. Bend your knees in and exhale, using your abdominals to draw the knees and chest toward each other and then lower down again. Repeat eight times. Do two sets.

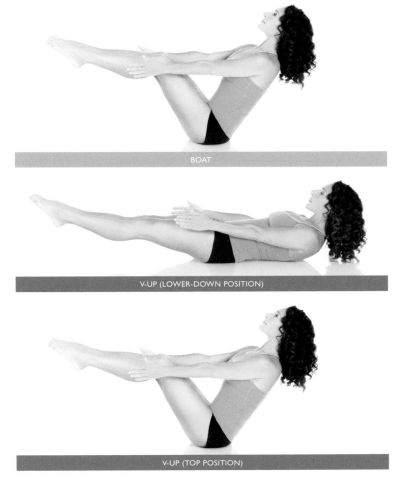

BOAT

V-UP (LOWER-DOWN POSITION)

V-UP (TOP POSITION)

## CONNECT (MEDITATION)

Sit in a comfortable cross-legged position, ideally with your hips above your knees. You may also have the option of sitting in a chair with both feet planted on the floor. Place the tops of your hands on your knees so that your palms are open. Extend out through the crown of your head. Meditation is mindful breathing, so simply place your awareness on your breath. You can try inhaling on a four-count and holding for two and then exhaling on a six-count. Notice your connection to the universe, the physical sensation, and the feelings arising as you sit in your place.

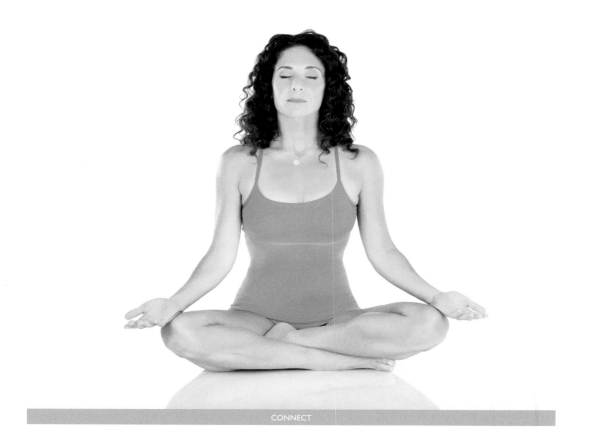

CONNECT

# FOOD PLAN

**W**hether your goal is to lose weight or simply get more toned and aligned with your body, healthy eating habits are critical to the Yogalosophy program. Why? Because food affects the way you feel. Food has consciousness. So when you eat, every human and circumstance that had contact with what you are consuming gets incorporated into your cells and actually becomes a part of you. When you opt for clean foods, not only will you feel healthier and more energized, but you will also experience a greater sense of clarity, and cultivate a more grounded, centered foundation to come from throughout your day. Most important is the attitude with which you eat your food. So keep in mind that whatever you choose to eat, enjoy it and eat it wholeheartedly.

The Yogalosophy Diet Plans are varied, but they all work very well. My suggestion is that you choose one of the three options and stick with it, instead of bouncing from one to the next. Your body needs a chance to adapt, and if you keep switching around, you will not reap the same rewards. In order to see results, choose the Diet Plan you know you can stick with.

The purpose of the next twenty-eight days is to commit to a plan that works for you and go through that process. There are many, many ways to eat, and I have tried most of them. There's no "right way." Consider it an experiment and try to have fun with it! You will lose weight as a byproduct. I promise!

## OPTION A: *Clean*

This option is best for those of you who want to focus on portion control without having to give up meat, dairy, and grains. I have had great luck with eating small amounts of dense foods and feeling satiated because I am not depriving myself.

## OPTION B: *Lean*

I developed a loose version of a yeast-free diet. This plan is challenging and focuses on eliminating grains and foods that break down into sugars. The beauty of this diet is its lack of caloric restriction, so I eat tons of avocado and nuts and still end up losing weight. I also feel amazing when I get off of sugars because it balances out my insulin levels.

## OPTION C: *Green*

I grew up vegan, so I have experience eating a plant-based diet. This is the one to try if you are vegan, or even if you are vegan-curious. Nothing feels better than being dairy-free! This plan includes grains and legumes. You will be amazed how tasty you will find your living foods.

## EATING GUIDELINES

You will find complete recipes and menus for each diet plan beginning on page 242, but here are the basic guidelines:

- Eat whole foods that are as close to their natural state as possible. Try always to select organic, clean foods that are not GMO. Many food allergies and physical problems are due to nonlabeled genetically modified foods in our food supply, so do your research. If it doesn't say non-GMO or organic, assume it is not.

- Do not eat any packaged, processed foods. If it's in a package, you want to avoid it.

- Cut out most sugars. The specifics will vary with each diet option, but in general the idea is not to put anything into your body that will spike your blood-sugar levels by metabolizing quickly. If you need something to sweeten your food, the natural sweetener stevia is ideal, but avoid all added sweeteners like evaporated cane juice (a.k.a., sugar!). The following sweeteners may be included in some recipes in moderation: honey, agave, and maple syrup.

- Eat breakfast. A protein breakfast is best, but there is some variety if you are following the vegan option. Make protein and vegetables the staple mainstay of your lunch, and make veggies the bulk of your dinner.

- Avoid caffeine. Do the best you can, opt for organic, and choose decaf. This is a tough one for me, but you will be amazed how good you feel. You can replace coffee with the less-caffeinated option, green tea, or entirely caffeine-free herbal teas.

- Hydrate. Drink at least sixty ounces of water (about two liters) a day.

By eating a fresh, plant-based, nutrient-packed diet and keeping your body hydrated, you make your body as receptive to change as possible—vibrant, whole foods encourage vitality. For each of the options, you get a grocery list and a week's sample meal plan. The goal is not to follow a rigid diet forever, but to teach you how to make healthy, slimming choices most of the time. If you are still hungry between meals, feel free to snack on anything on the "Yes" list for your option.

## OPTION A: *Clean*

This option is for the omnivore.

**YES:**

- Meat and poultry (organic and free-range whenever possible)
- Fish and shellfish
- Eggs
- Greek yogurt, kefir, parmesan cheese, and goat cheese
- All nonstarchy veggies: salad greens, celery, broccoli, cauliflower, spinach, eggplant, kale, collard greens, onions, peppers, tomatoes, mushrooms, asparagus, artichoke, zucchini, jicama, leeks, okra, etc.
- Nuts: almonds, cashews, pine nuts, pistachios, hazelnuts, macadamias, pecans, and walnuts
- Pumpkin and sunflower seeds
- Fats: olive oil, coconut oil, avocado, and olives
- Condiments: balsamic vinegar, mustard, soy sauce, Braggs Liquid Aminos
- Berries, fruits of all kinds

**NO:**

- Alcohol
- Sugars
- Artificial sweeteners

**WHAT A TYPICAL DAY EATING THIS WAY LOOKS LIKE:**

- **BREAKFAST:** Mushroom omelet with avocado slices
- **MIDMORNING SNACK:** handful of cashews
- **LUNCH:** Sautéed salmon with large salad of field greens with balsamic vinaigrette, walnuts, and olives
- **AFTERNOON SNACK:** Celery stalks with almond butter
- **DINNER:** Grilled eggplant, zucchini, tomato, and asparagus with chicken breast

CLEAN

## OPTION B: *Lean*

This is a lacto-ovo vegetarian option.

**YES:**

- Eggs
- Tofu and tempeh
- Greek yogurt, kefir, parmesan cheese, and goat cheese
- All nonstarchy veggies: salad greens, celery, broccoli, cauliflower, spinach, eggplant, kale, collard greens, onions, peppers, tomatoes, mushrooms, artichoke, zucchini, jicama, leeks, okra, etc.
- Nuts: almonds, cashews, pine nuts, pistachios, hazelnuts, macadamias, pecans, and walnuts
- Pumpkin and sunflower seeds
- Fats: olive oil, coconut oil, avocado, and olives
- Condiments: balsamic vinegar, mustard, soy sauce, Braggs Liquid Aminos

**NO:**

- Fruit
- Potatoes, yams, sweet potatoes
- Grains
- Alcohol
- Sugars
- Artificial sweeteners

**WHAT A TYPICAL DAY EATING THIS WAY LOOKS LIKE:**

- **BREAKFAST:** Veggie omelet
- **MIDMORNING SNACK:** Greek yogurt with cinnamon
- **LUNCH:** Spinach salad with tomatoes, goat cheese, walnuts, olives, and balsamic vinaigrette
- **AFTERNOON SNACK:** Ice-blended almond shake
- **DINNER:** Grilled eggplant, zucchini, tomato, and asparagus with tempeh

LEAN

## OPTION C: *Green*

This is a vegan choice.

**YES:**

- Beans and other legumes (peas, etc.)
- Tofu and protein replacements (make sure they are non-GMO, as many soy products have been genetically modified)
- Grains: corn, brown rice, quinoa
- Yams
- Berries, grapefruit, apples
- All types of veggies
- Nuts: almonds, cashews, pine nuts, pistachios, hazelnuts, macadamias, pecans, and walnuts
- Pumpkin and sunflower seeds
- Fats: olive oil, coconut oil, avocado, and olives
- Condiments: balsamic vinegar, mustard, soy sauce, Braggs Liquid Aminos

**NO:**

- Meats
- Dairy
- Alcohol
- Sugars (other than the fruits listed in the "Yes" column)
- Artificial sweeteners

**WHAT A TYPICAL DAY EATING THIS WAY LOOKS LIKE:**

- **BREAKFAST:** Hemp protein shake with blueberries
- **MIDMORNING SNACK:** Handful of almonds, or almond butter on apple slices
- **LUNCH:** Kale and white bean soup and an enormous salad (cabbage, arugula, tomato, avocado, pecans, olives, radishes, etc.)
- **AFTERNOON SNACK:** Half an avocado drizzled with olive oil and salt
- **DINNER:** Veggie stir-fry with tofu

GREEN

# PART 2

# The Y28 Revolution

# DAY 1

## SET INTENTION
### *Name It to Claim It*

I want to let you in on a little secret: You already have a design and a potential within you that wants to take root and come to fruition. The way you begin something has a great effect on the outcome. I know this from experience; I have never had a dream that did not come true. I have also never had a fear that didn't come true. So the question you need to ask yourself is, What do you want to create?

Every single thing that exists started out as an idea. When you realize how powerful your intentions are, that those seeds you are planting with your beliefs actually grow, you can claim your birthright as a creator. You can actually re-create your body and your mind and have what you want through your intention! Intention sets the tone for the way you start something and has the greatest effect on its outcome. One of the all-time great takeaways from yoga is the power of setting intention. I do this at the beginning of the yoga practice. It can be a dedication, a point of focus, or simply the lens through which you would like to see throughout the practice—and beyond. You can bring this yoga philosophy, or Yogalosophy, into everything you do. That goes for the way you start your day, the way you begin a project, the moment when you sit down to eat a meal.

> *"Whatever you can do or dream you can do, begin it. Boldness has genius, power, and magic in it. Begin it now."*
>
> — GOETHE

Think of yourself as a flower or a tree. The seed of potential is within you, and the way you cultivate this seed has a great effect on how that design will grow and unfold. For instance, if you did not water and feed it, it would likely wither and die. More importantly, if you plant an apple seed, no matter what you do, you will not be able to turn that apple tree into a pumpkin patch. So you must also become very honest and authentic about what type of a seedling you are and what you should expect from yourself as you grow into yourself.

Let me tell you how setting intention has affected my life. Right before I started teaching, I was going through a major transitional phase. My former career had come to a standstill, and I was unsure how I was going to leap into the next phase of my life. I had a faint idea in the back of my mind that I would be sharing myself with others on a public and personal level. I was not sure how, as I had been directionless for five years. After a career as a young actress, an eating disorder, my parents' divorce, the loss of a dear friend to a shooting, and my own random physical assault, I was thawing out. I was no longer the same person I had been before. My tree had been shaken to its roots. It seemed like a much-needed break at first, but what started out as respite had become a slump. I had been jobless and living off the money I had made in my youth; however, that was dwindling down. It became a matter of survival to find my new form of employment.

I would have done anything, and I did try a few jobs on for size. I packed someone for their move, I was a personal assistant to a writer, I cast an industrial film, and I put out the word that I would do any type of work. I did not realize that saying it out loud would open the door to an even more rewarding, brand new life. I had several healing sessions with my therapist, who asked me to define my personal mission statement, which was: "Integrate all facets of myself in order to inspire self-love." In all honesty, I knew that this was a tall order. Integrate ALL facets of myself? Inspire self-love in others? Did I even love myself? How would I inspire it in others? Integrating my opposing energies seemed impossible at the time. But there it was. I said it. I declared my intention.

Shortly, very shortly, say two weeks after that, I was offered a job teaching spinning (indoor cycling) classes at a Santa Monica studio that was just opening. I said yes. I said yes to anything at that time. Of course, I was terrified that first day I was asked to teach among the other twelve teachers who had opened the studio. They had all been my teachers and mentors for years, and I was the chubby student in the corner wearing seven layers of sweat clothes with my nose buried in a book between classes so that I wouldn't have to look at myself in the mirror or speak to anyone. I was overweight and antisocial, unlike any exercise instructor I had ever seen.

We all arrived in the former dance studio and the owner asked us to go around and declare what our intention was for this adventure. When it came to me, I shyly blurted, "I would like to share with others what I have been given and what I have learned." Little did I know what a powerful statement this was!

Within fifteen days, many of the teachers who I had compared myself to lost interest and left the studio. There weren't enough students for them to stay motivated. But I hung in there and did what my mentor at the time told me to do: speak out loud what you say to yourself when you are exercising. *I couldn't do that,* I thought. Surely people would think I was insane! Those thoughts in my head were mine alone. No one else would understand me. Well I kept waking up each day and declaring my intention, to share and to give as much of myself, and make each class the best I ever taught. I kept sharing my inner voice. Not the self-doubter. Sure, I'd bring her into the picture. She was a bit of an attention seeker, so if I didn't give her the stage she would steal scenes. But my best self was allowed the forum. And she was great.

The response was surprising. At first I had trouble making even $30 a week, but I continued to give and to open my heart and my mouth, while holding my intention as a seedling in the back of my mind. At the end of twenty-eight days, my class had grown from three to thirty people. The studio owner needed to order more bikes because of my classes. Within three months, I talked her into allowing me to teach two classes. When she asked me to let go of my 7:00 AM time slot to allow a more seasoned teacher to fill it, I said okay and taught 8:00 AM instead, which consequently became packed. Within nine months, I was teaching to one hundred people, with fifty on my waiting list daily. I was named "Best Of" in *Los Angeles* magazine, and the students flocked to my class. Oh, and on a sidenote, my body fell right into place, naturally.

I believe that people were attracted to my class because I stuck to my intention. Not only did I become the most celebrated spinning teacher in Los Angeles, where celebrities and cancer survivors, athletes and studio execs would come to get their catharsis on and that extra layer off, I had planted the seed for the much larger intention that I had originally set for myself. I was beginning to integrate all facets of myself in order to inspire self-love. I would not have imagined that a mere decade later, I would become a public figure, an expert in the field of manifesting my best life via the journey of the body. And now I am sharing that here with you. You can have what I have. It does not matter what you weigh, whether or not you are in love or have money or enough time. Whatever you have is perfect as is, and you do not have to wait. Begin it now!

## START WHERE YOU ARE

The very best way to make a change toward getting the life you want is by putting yourself into physical action. Believe it or not, every goal that you have for your life begins in your body. Exercise and physical movement have a way of reorganizing your cells. In fact, a recent study conducted in Sweden explains how exercise changes your DNA. Researchers were able to measure how the muscles read the blueprint of your physical body during high-intensity exercise. Thus a shift in the way that your body takes shape! Imagine all of the immeasurable changes that also occur on a mental, emotional, and even psychic level during an exercise session.

All parts of my life tend to sync up when I am exercising. I have often been surprised that life resolves itself while I am in a class. I have had life-changing epiphanies, creative surges, and problem resolutions while in midsweat. I get the phone call I have been waiting for, or a better offer comes through during that hour I took for myself.

## NAME IT TO CLAIM IT

In order to have what you want, you must name it. Say what you want out loud. Write it down, and allow yourself to be seen and heard. More importantly, see and believe it yourself. Declare your intention. Naming and declaring what you want is extremely powerful. It is literally like your own magic spell or incantation. Beginning your yoga practice with an intention brings meaning to your workout that exceeds your body or the shape of your tush (although that counts too!). It starts the ball rolling. Many of us adopt a superstitious attitude regarding saying what we want. We are taught to believe that it's selfish. Some of us do not want to be disappointed, so never call it, for fear that the outcome will not go as planned. If you are concerned you will make the wrong decision, well hey, you can just dump it and start all over again. Until you go for it, you just never know what might occur along the way. And guess what? Once you get what you want, there will be another thing right around the corner. So don't get too attached to the outcome!

I believe that desire is God-given, and that following that impulse is using your intuition. It will lead you to the correct place. Be a leader. Be an inspiration and declare yourself!

## ACTION CHECKLIST

### INTENTION: *Be selfish!*

Ask yourself what you want, and declare it. Claim your power, name it, and connect with it at the beginning of your routine, as well as throughout the day.

### PLAYLIST: *Start Me Up*

This is a list of some of my favorite songs to pump myself up with. For your cardio bursts today, choose one of mine, or pick one of your own.

"Start Me Up," Rolling Stones
"Respect," Aretha Franklin
"Hopeless Place," Rihanna
"Let's Go Crazy," Prince
"Connected," Stereo MCs
"Good Vibrations," Marky Mark
"Higher Love," Steve Winwood
"Life Is A Highway," Tom Cochrane
"One More Time," Daft Punk
"Ramble On," Led Zeppelin

### YOGALOSOPHY ROUTINE VARIATION

See pages 9 through 24 for this main routine. It's the staple of your workout plan, but there will be daily changes. Start with two sets of each yoga/toner combo. Hold each pose for five to eight breaths. Do eight reps, plus eight pulses, of each toner.

### CARDIO OPTION

Choose a song that gets you fired up and play it four times today while doing the exercises listed below. These five-minute bursts will add up to twenty minutes of cardio, and you will burn calories just by having fun! I suggest the following moves, but feel free to play around with it:

Do each move for one minute:

- Jumping Jacks
- Forward kicks
- Side kicks
- Knee lifts
- Running in place

Remember to listen to your body. These are the day's suggestions. If you don't get it at first, be positive and listen to your body's cues.

DAY 1

# POSE OF THE DAY

## BOAT POSE WITH AB LEG EXTENSIONS

(See photos on next page for pose demonstration.)

Balance on your sit bones. Start with your feet up and knees bent so that your calves are parallel to the floor. Extend your arms forward, parallel to the floor with palms facing each other, and lift your chest and sternum upward. Press your shoulders down as you gaze up. Then extend your legs straight so that your toes are at eye level. Balance here, using your lower abdominal muscles. Imagine pressing your lower back forward as you lift your chest upward toward the ceiling. Slowly lower both the upper and lower body down and hover your shoulders and feet a few inches off the floor, arms extended and hovering as well, straight along your sides. Draw your right knee in, and then extend the right leg straight up. Keep the leg straight as you lower it down alongside the left leg. Switch sides, raising the left leg. One more time each side, then sweep back into Boat Pose with the knees bent. Finally, extend the legs straight, coming into Full Boat. Hold for two breaths.

Connect to your sense of identity, willpower, and desire. Follow your gut. Boat Pose connects you to the center point of your body, where your original cell is. An inch in and two inches below the navel center is the place where you were connected to your mother when you were just being formed. Reconnect to this place to align with your sense of self.

PHYSICAL BENEFITS: Abdominal muscle toning, great for building core strength.

HEALING BENEFITS: Helps aid digestion, generates heat in the body.

EMOTIONAL ASPECTS: Connects us to our individual identity, desire, and awareness of what we want. Strengthens our willpower.

MODIFICATIONS: For an easier version, you can bend your knees or support yourself by placing your hands on the floor behind you.

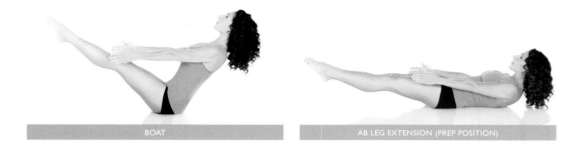

BOAT

AB LEG EXTENSION (PREP POSITION)

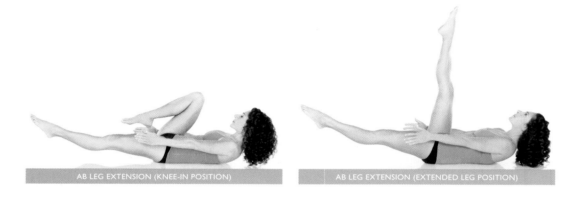

AB LEG EXTENSION (KNEE-IN POSITION)

AB LEG EXTENSION (EXTENDED LEG POSITION)

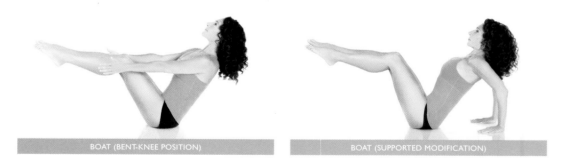

BOAT (BENT-KNEE POSITION)

BOAT (SUPPORTED MODIFICATION)

## EXTRA CREDIT: *Get prepared!*

Set an intention for this twenty-eight-day program. Choose a diet plan. Go food shopping.

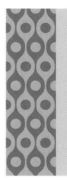

■ **DIET MODIFICATION:** *Week 1*

- Choose the diet option that you feel is right for you.
- Eliminate refined, processed, and packaged foods.
- Choose organic whole foods: fresh fruits and vegetables.
- Increase your water intake: Drink a minimum of two liters of water per day.

## Recipe: SMOOTHIE
### (WILL WORK FOR ANY DIET OPTION)

Smoothies are so easy to make. They can be a meal replacement or a snack, and they are a yummy treat, packed with nutrients.

**1 cup almond milk**
**1 cup frozen berries**
**1 cup purified water**
**1 tablespoon almond butter or tahini**
**1 small packet (⅛ teaspoon) stevia**

Toss in a blender until liquefied. Drink.

# DAY 2

## MAKE SHORT-TERM GOALS

### *See the Finish Line*

The beauty of setting and reaching short-term goals is that you get immediate gratification, which gives your brain positive reinforcement. Everyone responds to doing well. When we achieve a goal, we feel a sense of victory. That feeling is a reward in itself. How many of us make the mistake of saying right up front, "I need to lose twenty pounds"? That type of goal is just too lofty and far away and can be discouraging when you don't see immediate results. That's why I believe in short-term goals for sustained results. Little markers and milestones along the way will help to remind you that you are on the right track. Setting yourself up with little wins is like having a built-in cheering section.

> *"Warriors jump over walls, they don't demolish them."*
>
> — CARLOS CASTANEDA

Think of each day in this book as a goalpost. Think only of the action tasks of the day. You can easily make a change for a single day, right? Each day, begin again and start fresh, just like a child. Before you know it, these short-term goals you accomplish will bring you across the finish line.

I remember a game my brother and I would play when we were children. Our goal was to get to the local store and buy a treat. The two-hour uphill walk seemed like an endless journey, so we created different landmarks along the way. The reservoir view. The house with the Jack Russell puppy. My Aunt Gertrude's yellow house. I would play these mental games with myself just to stay the course. There were moments on that hike through the hills where I wanted to quit, but eventually it was just too late to give up. So I would try skipping or hopping on one leg to the next signpost. Sometimes my brother, Dave, and I would compete with a quick sprint to the next stop sign or collaborate on a funny song about our parents. These baby steps felt like small victories and kept us going. Ultimately we would reach our goal. The reason it felt so good was because we built up to it. Now I'm here to tell you: You can do it too!

## SEE THE FINISH LINE

Any goal that I have ever reached started with an intention, but it had to be reinforced by a picture in my mind. When I would begin that trek to the local grocery store, I would start by closing my eyes and imagining myself at the market destination at the top of that hill, sipping a cold soda. (It was the early '70s; we didn't know any better!) It began in my mind's eye before it became reality. The eye likes to have a visual image to connect with the tangible result. The eye delights in images that motivate and inspire—something that can be seen.

This is why each year I encourage my students to create a vision board that connects them with their hopes and dreams. (I'll share how you can make your own later in this chapter.) This is a poster board where you can arrange a collage of images that represents all areas of your life: personal life, how you look, finances, possessions, your neighborhood, family, home, leisure, children, creative projects, work, health, being of service, relationships, love, business, death, transformation and the shadow side, travel, education, spirituality, career, and who you are in the world, friendships, community, spirituality, and the unknown. The vision board should have all of this and more. Phrases that motivate you, deadlines, inspiring quotes, drawings, or personal pictures. . . . You get the idea!

I actually made my vision board into a Vision Yoga Mat! Where better to be inspired than while I am practicing yoga? The images on my yoga mat motivate me and permeate my DNA with inspired feeling! Looking back, it's as if my last couple of years are right there on that visual map.

## ✕ ACTION CHECKLIST

**INTENTION:** *Beginner's mind*

Be like a child. When you start from a place of not knowing, the world of possibility and discovery will open up to you. Each day you wake up, you have a new body, a new opportunity to explore in a different way. When you come to your yoga practice with a beginner's mind, you can open up to the present moment and what is happening now. Be open and teachable today.

**PLAYLIST:** *Sweet Child o' Mine*

When you listen to music you heard as a child, it can take you right back to that beginner's mind. Here is a playlist of some of my favorite songs from childhood. You can use mine or create your own.

"Beautiful Child," Fleetwood Mac

"Sunshine On My Shoulders," John Denver

"Let's Stay Together," Al Green

"Honky Cat," Elton John

"Coconut," Harry Nilsson

"My Sweet Lord," George Harrison

"The Air That I Breathe," The Hollies

"Moonlight Mile," Rolling Stones

"Wild Horses," Rolling Stones

"Going to California," Led Zeppelin

"Never Can Say Goodbye," Jackson 5

"Landslide," Fleetwood Mac

"Come Down in Time," Elton John

**YOGALOSOPHY ROUTINE VARIATION**

After two sets of the Yogalosophy routine, reward yourself with a one-minute cardio interval. (See below for options.) Think of each exercise in the routine as a milestone. When we have a goal for ourselves, it may not always be clear or logical how we will get there. More will be revealed. "I don't know" is a very powerful stance to take. See if you can take this attitude with you throughout your workout and into your day.

**CARDIO OPTION:** *Some interval options*

- Run in place
- Jumping jacks
- Knee kicks
- Side kicks
- Jumping side to side
- Hopping
- Skipping
- Jumping twists
- Forward kicks
- Side to side stepping
- Jumping lunges
- Dancing

DAY 2

## POSES OF THE DAY

### Warrior 2, Reverse Warrior, Side Angle Pose

Isn't it interesting that yoga is stereotypically associated with peace and love, hippies and pacifists, yet many poses are versions of Warrior? Explore what it means to embody the stance and energy of a warrior. The term *hatha yoga* means "the yoga of force." If you avoid this fierceness, you become lazy and lose focus. Don't be afraid of feeling strong, even "fierce." It's a very powerful and motivating force. You can channel that right into exercise and assume the position: Act like a warrior!

Add these poses in after the lunges and before Temple in the Yogalosophy routine.

### WARRIOR 2

Stand with your feet wide apart. Turn your right toes out to the right, and line your right heel with the arch of your left (back) foot. Bend your right (front) knee to a ninety-degree angle. Extend your arms out to shoulder level and gaze down the center of your right hand. Your shoulders, hips, and knees should be in alignment. Imagine two pieces of clear glass pressing in on both sides of you, sandwiching you in between. Your gaze is fixed and pointed down the center of your hand past your fingertips. Your aim is clear, and you become alert, relaxed, confident, and focused. Take five to ten deep breaths. Move to . . .

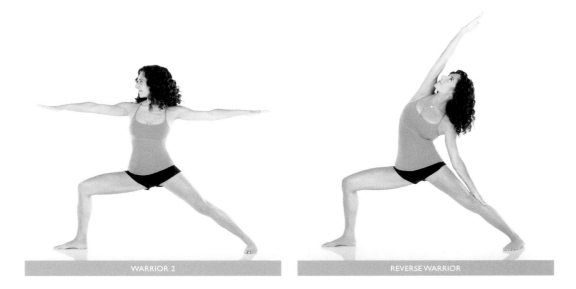

WARRIOR 2      REVERSE WARRIOR

## REVERSE WARRIOR

Slide your left (back) hand down the left hamstring as you extend your right arm up and over. Align your biceps with your cheek. Take five to ten deep breaths. Return to Warrior 2.

## SIDE ANGLE POSE

Bring your right (front) forearm onto the right thigh. Pressing away from the thigh will create more space and elongate the neck. Extend the left arm up and over. Take five to ten deep breaths. Return to Warrior 2 and repeat on left side.

**PHYSICAL BENEFITS:** Tones and strengthens legs, stretches hamstrings and groin.

**HEALING BENEFITS:** Brings blood flow to the joints and burns calories.

**EMOTIONAL ASPECTS:** Strengthens determination and focus, aids in moving forward.

**MODIFICATIONS:** If you have sensitive knees, do not bend to ninety degrees. Instead, straighten your front leg and shorten your stance to a Triangle Pose (see page 58). For a deeper stretch, bring your hand to the floor.

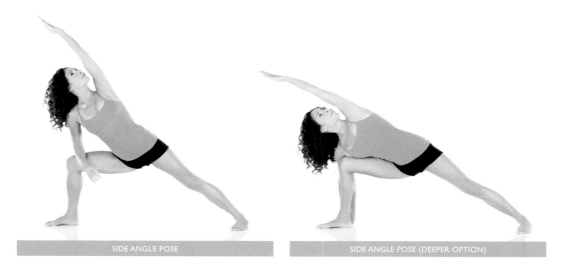

SIDE ANGLE POSE          SIDE ANGLE POSE (DEEPER OPTION)

# EXTRA CREDIT: *Create a vision board.*

You can make your board on a piece of poster board and hang it somewhere inspirational, or you can have your vision imposed onto a yoga mat, like I did.

## MATERIALS YOU WILL NEED:

- Poster board
- Magazines
- Photos
- Colored markers
- Yellow highlighter
- Glue stick
- Personal photos
- Glitter, sequins, or anything else you can think of!

## INSTRUCTIONS FOR CREATING YOUR VISION BOARD

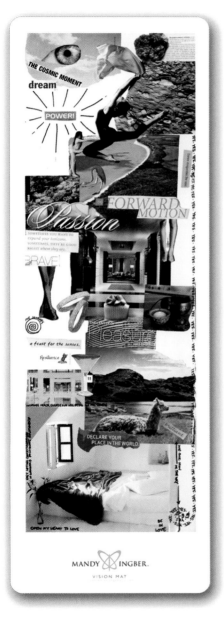

1 Begin by outlining the entire poster board in yellow with your highlighter. Yellow is the color associated with the third chakra at the center of the body. Imagine a spinning wheel of energy behind your belly button. It directly connects you with your willpower, desire, and identity. Marking your board with this colored marker declares to the universe: This is what I want!

2 Tear out or cut out all the images that you love and that speak to you. I like to include lots of pictures from nature and the cosmos. Travel magazines, National Geographic, and magazines with lots of pictures work very well.

3 Arrange your collage in any way you like.

**4** Glue your images to the board.

**5** Add any writings and layer your vision board in any way that pleases you.

**6** If you like, add the date, title it, or put your mission statement on it.

**7** Place it somewhere that you will see it. Your subconscious mind will absorb it.

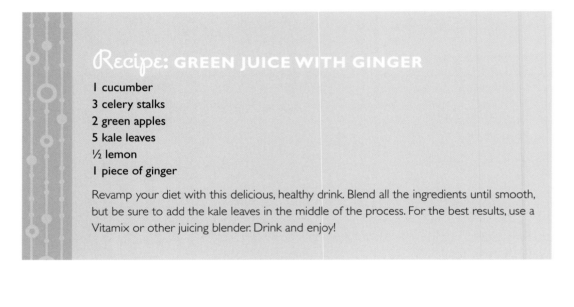

*Recipe:* **GREEN JUICE WITH GINGER**

1 cucumber
3 celery stalks
2 green apples
5 kale leaves
½ lemon
1 piece of ginger

Revamp your diet with this delicious, healthy drink. Blend all the ingredients until smooth, but be sure to add the kale leaves in the middle of the process. For the best results, use a Vitamix or other juicing blender. Drink and enjoy!

# DAY 3

## COME TO YOUR SENSES

### *Power Is in the Present Moment*

M any spiritual practices and guides encourage us to renounce our bodies and our senses. What if it's exactly the opposite? What if the most spiritual thing you can do is to become completely present to your senses? Although you may have been taught by your family, your religion, or society that there is something wrong with succumbing to them, your senses are a compass and they are where you connect with the power of the universe. Your seat of power is the present moment, and your senses are the tools to access this power.

The gifts of taste, touch, smell, sound, and sight are your birthright. These gifts are free and cannot be bought back if you lose them. Most of us possess nature's most awesome and valuable gifts and take them for granted.

*"Life is available only in the present moment. If you abandon the present moment you cannot live the moments of your daily life deeply."*

— THICH NHAT HANH

I know that I forget all the time what a miracle my body is, and how lucky I am to be in it for this brief time. I am constantly forgetting and reminding myself throughout the day. And then I forget again.

The greatest and most spiritual times I've ever experienced didn't happen in my head as an idea, but happened in my body as a felt sense. The simplicity of presence has such an awesome impact! For instance, right now I am sitting in my kitchen that looks out onto a sunlit mountain. I am listening to birds chirping and singing outside. There is an airplane I can hear flying overhead. I can feel the keys on my computer keyboard as I am tapping them. Even though I am wearing flannel, I feel a slight chill in the air. The roses on my table are a little bit old, so there is a funky flower smell wafting toward me, and I can faintly taste the remnants of tea tree oil toothpaste in my mouth. All that is impacting me at once—and it's all through my senses! Take a moment to sit where you are and notice what your senses are telling you. Just stop what you are doing for a moment. Take a breath. Come to your senses right now and notice how you feel.

I remember watching a television interview on PBS with Joseph Campbell. He is considered one of our greatest scholars, philosophers, and teachers, and he wrote the critically acclaimed book *The Power of Myth*. As he was speaking of spirituality and God, he shared that one of his most profound spiritual experiences happened while he was running on the beach at dusk. Wow, I thought. This is one of our great scholars, and even he uses the body and senses to connect with God. I knew exactly what he meant. Exercise gives you that powerful connection to the feeling of presence and immersion in the immediate moment. It requires that all of your energy gather to push you past an obstacle, and so it takes you right out of your head and into your body! I witness this when I watch a basketball game and an athlete makes a seemingly impossible shot that comes straight from being in the zone.

Today is a day to slow down enough to appreciate the energy of Mother Earth. A time to include the nurture of nature, appreciate the earthly plane, and remember that your body is but a manifestation of the spiritual. Be willing to indulge your senses, but notice what nourishes you and makes you feel grounded. Listen to your body for the messages it holds.

## ❧ ACTION CHECKLIST

**INTENTION:** *Pleasure.*

Come to your senses! Let your senses guide you through your day. Slow down and allow yourself to truly experience how wonderful it is to be able to fulfill your basic human needs. Engage the five senses.

**PLAYLIST:** *Mountain Climb*

I designed this spinning playlist to simulate a mountain climb. It was meant to be a gradual climb, and a resistance-loading challenge. This endurance ride is broken up with two one-minute sprints (one at the end of "Insomnia," and again during "Born Slippy"). Keep this in mind during your cardio workout.

"Before Today," Everything But the Girl

"Crash," Dave Matthews Band

"Find My Baby," Moby

"4 Minutes," Madonna

"Insomnia," Faithless

"Bitter Sweet Symphony," The Verve

"Kiss," Prince

"Bad," U2

"Born Slippy," Underworld

"September/The Joker," Fatboy Slim

"Sure Looks Good to Me," Alicia Keys

### YOGALOSOPHY ROUTINE VARIATION

Set the tone for your practice today by indulging your senses. Create a beautiful environment that is sensual and physically pleasing. Light a scented candle or some incense, swing the doors open to let in some fresh air, place flowers near your mat to beautify your practice, have a cool glass of water with cucumber or warm tea made with fresh mint, nearby. Anything that is physically pleasing to you will do.

Routine Modification: Skip the Yogalosophy toners, but hold the yoga half of the Yogalosophy postures for two minutes (or ten breaths). Breathe into it, and as you feel the burn, remember: It's not pain; it's just another sensation. Just be in it and feel it.

### CARDIO OPTION

Take a thirty- to sixty-minute walk or hike.

DAY 3

# POSE OF THE DAY

## TREE POSE

I chose Tree pose because a tree is one of the most beautiful things in nature, and for as tall as a tree grows, it must be equally rooted into the earth. Balance is about extending, so be sure to imagine the grounding force of pressing down into the earth. Imagine that you are being held inside of a tree trunk. Still, anchored, as you grow your arms wide open to the sky to receive. Committed to one spot. Feel your roots sinking deep into the earth.

Place most of your weight on your straight left leg and draw your right knee up and in toward your chest.

Extend up through your sternum and down through your straightened left leg.

Turn your right knee out as you bring the sole of your right foot to the inner thigh or calf of the left standing leg. Press the sole of your foot and the inner thigh together.

Steady your gaze and connect with your breathing.

Gently tuck your tailbone down toward your heel.

Press your palms together in prayer position at your heart, and then reach them up and over your head. Extend a line of energy out through the crown of the head as you connect with the midline running through the center of your body.

Hold for five to ten breaths and repeat on side two.

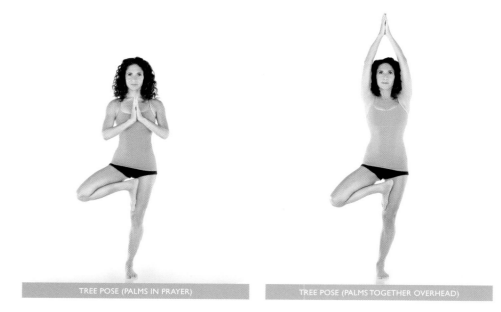

TREE POSE (PALMS IN PRAYER)

TREE POSE (PALMS TOGETHER OVERHEAD)

PHYSICAL BENEFITS: Tones thighs (inner), calves, and ankles. Stretches inner thigh, groin.

HEALING BENEFITS: Reduces sciatica, flat feet.

EMOTIONAL ASPECTS: Balance poses help us with patience and mental focus, and teach us preparation.

MODIFICATIONS: Bring sole of the foot to the ankle or calf. Use a wall or chair for balance.

## EXTRA CREDIT: *Taste it. Feel it. See it. Smell it. Listen to it.*

### TASTE IT.

Indulge! It's not the one bite of cake that you taste that causes weight gain. It's what you eat consistently that counts. I am a chocolate lover. My favorite is Zen Bunni dairy-free raw chocolate. Sea salt flavor. Yum. As long as I allow myself this indulgence occasionally, there is less backlash. Another way to treat your taste buds is to savor the flavor of nature. A trip to the farmers' market makes me feel so alive. I run a mental reminder in my head: "I am nature eating nature. God eating God." Enjoy natural flavors today. My favorite healthy treat is ripe avocado, sliced in half with pink salt. For a sweet treat: Pink Lady apple sprinkled with salt and cinnamon. I am also a big fan of mint tea with honey.

### FEEL IT.

We all need touch. The body craves it. There is no greater comfort than human warmth in the form of a hug or resting your head on the shoulder of a loved one. Another great way to pamper is with massage. If you cannot afford to schedule one, then trade with a friend. . . . You scratch their back and vice versa. Even your practice can serve as a self-massage. Yoga is not only for the muscles, joints, tendons, and ligaments. It also massages the internal organs as well. Have a snuggly blanket handy to swaddle yourself in at the end of your practice.

### SEE IT.

Beauty is very important for inner peace. What you see outside of you reflects the qualities within you. Start from the outside in. Practice with your vision board in the room today, so that your gaze can fall upon images that stimulate and inspire you. Some other options: choose flowers, objects from nature, or art to enhance your space.

## SMELL IT.

Scents can induce very powerful physical and emotional responses. Aromatherapy calms, energizes, and tones. Slather on vanilla oil, light some Naag Champa incense, or burn your favorite scented candle.

## LISTEN TO IT.

Music has always inspired me, and I am sure that you have sounds that inspire you. Explore the effects of sound on your practice. Try playing something uplifting and light. My current favorites:

**CLASSIC ROCK:** "Into the Mystic," Van Morrison

**CLASSICAL:** Fazil Say playing Bach

**CHANTING:** "Breath of the Heart," Krishna Das

**SOUNDS OF NATURE:** "Storm of Prayers," Shaman's Dream

## *Recipe:* MANDALAY MINI VACAY

Justin Theroux created this afternoon pick-me-up that satisfies all the senses and is rich in antioxidants (and all-around awesomeness!).

1 apple
2 squares dark chocolate
5 walnuts
¼ teaspoon cinnamon
Dash of cayenne
Sprinkle of salt
Handful of goji berries

Quarter and chop an apple. Dust with cinnamon, cayenne, and salt. Coarsely chop 2 squares of dark chocolate and 5 walnuts. Add ten to twenty goji berries. Arrange on a beautiful dish. Add a shot of espresso or mint tea with honey. Enjoy!

# DAY 4

## BE GRATEFUL

### *I Love What I Have, and I Want More!*

The first step to creating abundance is appreciating what you have. After all, if you can't appreciate what you already have, what makes you think you can appreciate more? It is essential to count your blessings and honor the gifts in your life on a daily basis.

When I was a little girl, I had a lack of gratitude. In fact, I felt perpetually disappointed. It seemed like no matter where I was, I felt dissatisfied. I was even unhappy with gifts that my mom gave me. The type of intimacy and connection I was looking for just didn't seem to exist, and I wasn't about to settle for what was happening in the moment. Even though I got good grades and passed tests with flying colors, I didn't feel smart. It was almost as if I was fooling everyone. I seemed to fit in with all of the groups at school, yet felt out of place.

> *"The roots of all goodness lie in the soil of appreciation for goodness."*
>
> — DALAI LAMA

I will never forget: There was a Christmas special that Johnny Carson did when I was a kid. For those of you who are too young to remember, Johnny Carson was the king of late-night shows before Jay Leno or David Letterman . . . or Jimmy Kimmel. He had a segment where he would read what kids wanted for Christmas, and I remember him reading a letter to Santa from one child who asked for a job for his dad. Another child had written that she wanted a jacket. It flattened me and brought me to tears. Even then, I had this awareness that within me was a lack of gratitude. I had a jacket. My father had a job. Why was I so demanding and dissatisfied? My tears did contain compassion for the children who had written, but primarily it was sadness, a shame that I took my blessings for granted.

I retrained my brain with something as simple as a gratitude list. Every day I make a list of five to ten things that I am grateful for, including things that don't necessarily seem like positives. When something happens that is out of my control, I put it at the top of my list. Something like getting fired or my breakup will have benefits that I cannot even imagine yet. So I have learned to put them at the top of my list as an act of faith. I don't expect you to do this, but it helps to cultivate a foundation of receptivity and acceptance. Experience has shown me that there are always gifts that come from these shake-ups.

The universe is continually gifting you with things. Some are simple as birds singing and the ability to take a deep breath, but sometimes the gifts are disguised in unfortunate circumstances. When my boyfriend left me, I did not know that the healing and self-loving I would do as a response would bring me a greater love, with new gifts. Or that losing my job would force me to use my yoga background and teaching skills to branch out and start to teach yoga. In my experience, everything is taken care of. So why not write a thank you card in advance?

With appreciation for your bounty of gifts in mind, it's time to add a gratitude list to your routine too—and that's exactly what you'll do today, along with some other gratefulness-inducing exercises.

As you think about what you will include in your gratitude list, remember that one of the greatest, most glorious gifts is your beautiful, capable, dare I say hot and sexy bod! Even if you're not so confident about your physique, believe me when I tell you there are many people out there who wish they had a body just like yours! So even if you're not your body's biggest fan, don't be afraid to add your "minuses" to your gratitude list. After all, what you focus on expands, and what could be better than becoming more and more grateful and appreciative of your body! Plus, studies show that cultivating contentment reduces your stress levels, which can result in weight loss and a positive shift in your responses. And finally, looking at your life through the lens of gratitude will allow you to have a better life, even if nothing changes. That's the whole point! Try adding true appreciation to your workout routine for the remainder of this program and watch your life get better.

## . . . AND I WANT MORE!

Yes, and! The old type of linear thinking says either/or, but in Yogalosophy we hold both at once. I love what I have AND I want more! It's important to know your value and value your needs. We are spiritual beings having a physical experience. It is okay to have possessions! Belongings are the physical manifestation of spirit. That's why I came up with the mantra: "I love what I have, and I want more!" It was not easy for me to admit this, as I was raised by a mother who had very little, and she learned to be satisfied with it.

My mother was the child of immigrants, so she was very poor growing up and never got into the habit of buying herself anything. I heard stories that she only had one doll, but when they had a toy drive at school, she was told she had to bring a toy to give to less fortunate children. What they didn't realize was that they were asking it of someone who had only one toy herself, and she didn't know how to communicate that she wanted to keep her doll. That feels like a sad story to me. To this day, my mother retains her belongings and even some of my past possessions. Of course, that means she has the original concert T-shirt from the Police Synchronicity tour, which I covet!

Although I appreciate her background, I had to learn that buying myself a gift is very healthy. If you need permission, I am giving you permission right now. Go out and buy yourself a gift today. Maybe a bouquet of flowers or a lotion that has your favorite scent. It doesn't have to be expensive, but magnify your appreciation of it. Savor it, and make it a gesture to the universe that you are grateful for what you have and are willing to accept more! Take good care of yourself and use your gift. Doesn't that feel great just imagining it? Think about it: When you give someone else a gift and you see them wearing it or using it, doesn't it make you feel good? One of the best ways to express gratitude for your gift is to use it, and that, my friend, is how happy the universe is when it witnesses you using your greatest gift: your body.

## FITNESS IS LIKE MONEY IN THE BANK

By putting a little bit away each day, you create security and can build ownership for yourself. Consider your exercise routine a deposit you are making every day into your health and well-being savings account. The Yogalosophy routine is like money in the bank and it adds up over time. Before you know it, you will have a wealth of health! Own your power and claim the richness of your birthright, which is your beautiful body.

## ✷ ACTION CHECKLIST

**INTENTION:** *Attitude of gratitude.*

Write out a list of five to ten things you feel grateful for. At least one must be about your physical body. Try to feel the gratitude instead of simply making a mental list. Include one thing that is challenging in your life today. Note that from here on out, creating a gratitude list will be part of your daily action. Be sure to include at least five gratitudes daily for the rest of the program.

Here's a list of things I am grateful for today:

- My freedom
- My toned legs
- Taking deep breaths
- Living near the ocean
- Sharing my process and helping others
- My sense of humor
- My ability to spin any situation to the positive

Now you try it.

### PLAYLIST: *Gratitude*

I use this playlist every Thanksgiving, and during the month of May. It's a great reinforcement to listen to songs that remind us to say "Thank You!"

"Gratitude," Earth, Wind & Fire

"Thank U," Alanis Morissette

"Thankful N' Thoughtful," Sly & The Family Stone

"Thank You," Christina Aguilera

"Be Thankful For What You've Got," Massive Attack

"Thank You," Sly & The Family Stone

"Thank You," Lil Bow Wow

"Thank You," Dido

"Fire On The Mountain," Grateful Dead

"Thank You," Led Zeppelin

"Thank You Boys," Jane's Addiction

"Thanks For The Information," Van Morrison

### YOGALOSOPHY ROUTINE VARIATION

New routine today! Replace the Yogalosophy routine with the grounding routine (see opposite page). Hold each posture for ninety seconds. Breathe through it and embrace the sensation.

### CARDIO OPTION

Take the same walk you took yesterday. Use all five of your senses as you experience your environment. Feel your way through it, and use it as a moving meditation. When you walk, the left and right hemispheres of the brain balance out. A walk is one of the healthiest and most natural activities you can do. Use all five of your senses as you experience your environment.

DAY 4

# GROUNDING ROUTINE

Chair Pose, Warrior 2, Triangle, Half Moon, Standing Splits, Standing Forward Bend, Squat, Cobbler's Pose, Pigeon, Seated Forward Bend

## CHAIR POSE

Stand with feet together. Remember your intention and take a deep breath in. Exhale. Sink your hips down, and as you sit into an imaginary chair, sweep your arms up overhead by your ears. Palms face each other. Shift your weight back toward your heels. Create as much space as you can between your shoulders and your ears. This pose is also called Lightning Bolt, so imagine lines of energy shooting out through your hands as well as down into the earth. Hold for ninety seconds (or ten slow breaths). Press yourself back up to standing and draw the palms into prayer position at your heart. Remind yourself one thing you are grateful for.

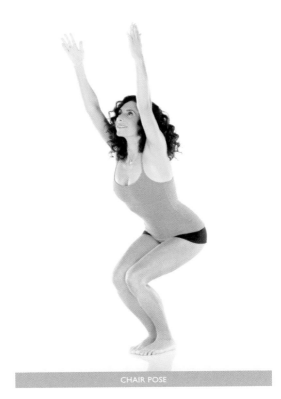

CHAIR POSE

## WARRIOR 2

Step your left foot back as far as you comfortably can. Turn your right foot out to the right and bend your right knee. Align your front (right) heel with your back (left) arch. Draw an imaginary line from the heel through the arch. Bend your front knee to a ninety-degree angle. Seal the outer edge of your left foot into the mat. Extend your arms out from the center of the body, reaching equally. Coax your right knee open, while the left ribs do the same to the left. Sink your hips down and reach your sternum up. Gaze down the center line of your hand (down toward your middle finger). Press the shoulders down, engaging the lateral muscles. Breathe. Pay particular attention to the grounded feeling of the lower body. Hold this for ten breaths or ninety seconds.

## TRIANGLE POSE

Straighten your front leg, and scooch the back foot in to narrow your stance. Shove your hips off to the left as you extend the right arm out to the right, reaching and elongating the underside of the torso. Place your right hand down on your shin, or if you are super flexible, alongside the outer edge of your right ankle. Extend the left arm up. Gaze upward. Try pressing the hips forward and leaning the upper body back so that your shoulders, hips, and feet are aligned. Breathe. Hold for ten breaths or ninety seconds.

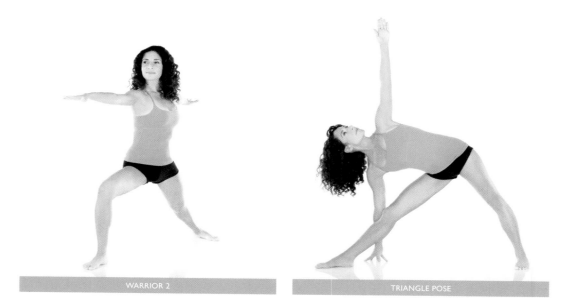

WARRIOR 2　　　　　　　　　　TRIANGLE POSE

## HALF MOON POSE

From Triangle, lower your extended top (left) hand to your hip as you launch into this balancing pose. Looking down toward the floor will help you stay grounded. Bend your front (right) leg and place your right fingertips on the floor, slightly off to the side in front of you. Shift your weight completely to the standing leg, and extend the left leg out behind you. Once you have your balance, stack your hips, reach up with your top arm, and hold. If you are wobbly, you can use a wall or a chair to support you. After ten breaths, lower the top hand to the floor.

## STANDING SPLITS

With both hands now on the floor on either side of the right foot, extend your sternum down toward the top of the foot. Your right leg should be straight while your left extended leg is lifted. Two schools of thought: one is to keep both hip bones aiming to the floor, and the other to open the hips as you raise the leg. Choose one. Be confident. Breathe. Hold for ten breaths.

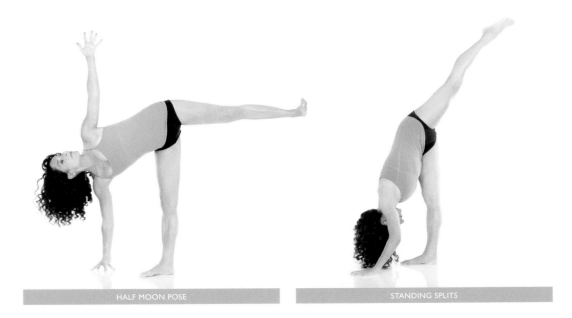

HALF MOON POSE                    STANDING SPLITS

## STANDING FORWARD BEND

Lower your leg to the floor and place both feet parallel, about hip-width apart. Hinge from your hips and allow the crown of your head to hang toward the floor. Just dangle down. You can shake the head "no" to release any tension that you may be holding in the neck, but simply breathe and be slow. Connect and ground through the feet down into the earth. You are completely supported, so just feel that and notice yourself slowing down. Hold for ninety seconds

Roll up to standing and repeat the first six poses on the left side.

## SQUAT

From a Standing Forward Bend, lower your hips down to a squat. Turn your toes out slightly. Bring your palms together in prayer position at the heart. You can use your elbows to gently press on the inner thighs and open your knees. If your heels do not come to the floor, try widening your stance, or you can roll up a small towel to place below your heels. Allow the hips to sink down, extend out through the crown of your head, and feel the natural traction that occurs while you are in this posture. Hold for ten breaths or ninety seconds.

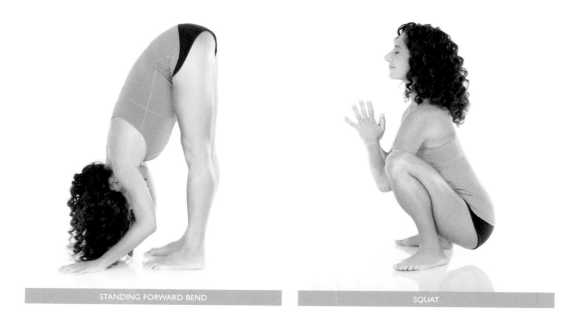

STANDING FORWARD BEND | SQUAT

## COBBLER'S POSE

Lower your hips all the way to the mat and place the soles of your feet together as your knees fan out to the sides. Hold onto your feet or ankles and grow tall through your spine. Take a deep breath in, and on the exhale draw your chest forward and down, hold, and breathe. After ninety seconds, come up to sitting.

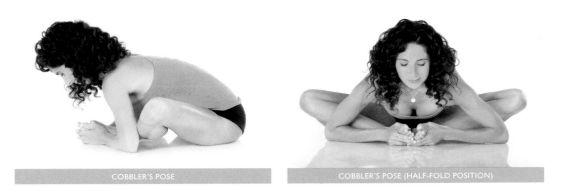

COBBLER'S POSE        COBBLER'S POSE (HALF-FOLD POSITION)

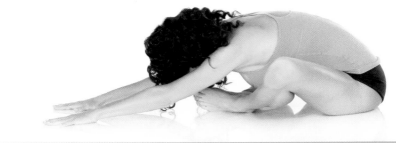

COBBLER'S POSE (FULL-FOLD POSITION)

From Cobbler's Pose, shift your weight to the right and, keeping the right leg bent, swing the left leg straight behind you. Square the hips to the floor. Your left knee should be directed toward the floor and both hips should be level. When you are ready, lower your torso down and settle here for ninety seconds. Walk the hands back and raise your body up. Switch sides. (If you have any knee issues, see the modification of this pose, Reclining Pigeon, on page 180.)

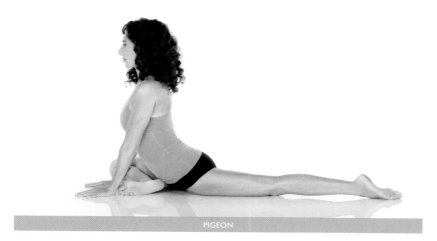

PIGEON

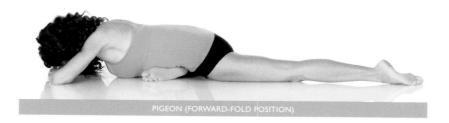

PIGEON (FORWARD-FOLD POSITION)

## SEATED FORWARD BEND

From Pigeon, swing your back leg forward and then extend both legs straight out in front of you. Move the fleshy part of the tush to the side so you are grounded on your sit bones. Extend and elongate the spine by imagining a line through the top of your head. Inhale and sweep the arms up overhead, and on the exhale, extend your sternum toward the tops of the feet and lower your chest down toward your legs. Breathe and stay here for ninety seconds.

You may modify this pose by using a strap to wrap around your feet if you cannot reach them.

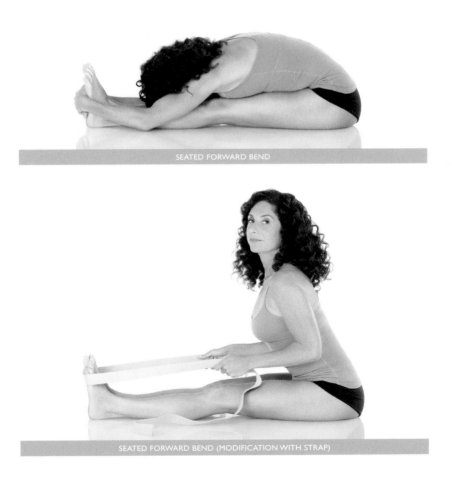

SEATED FORWARD BEND

SEATED FORWARD BEND (MODIFICATION WITH STRAP)

## POSE OF THE DAY

MOUNTAIN POSE

Standing with feet together, drop the tailbone down, aiming toward your heels. Roll the shoulders back and down. Feel a line of energy extending out through the crown of your head, and ground through the feet. Cover as much territory with your feet as possible so that you feel grounded at your base. Bring your palms together at your heart and say one thing you are grateful for about your body. (For example, "I am grateful that I can breathe" or "I am grateful that I am strong enough to stand.") Mountain Pose is the foundation of all other poses in hatha yoga.

PHYSICAL BENEFITS: Strengthens knees, thighs, and ankles; firms abs and tush; improves posture.

HEALING BENEFITS: Brings the focus internal.

EMOTIONAL ASPECTS: Helps you to become centered and grounded. This can cultivate self-reliance.

MODIFICATIONS: Stand with feet apart to decrease intensity.

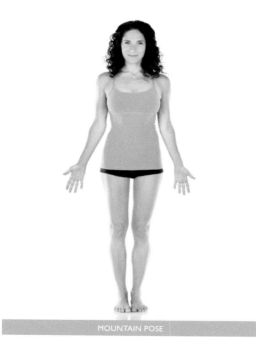

MOUNTAIN POSE

## EXTRA CREDIT: *Treat yourself!*

Buy yourself a gift, or take some time to get a massage or a beauty treatment. Indulge yourself.

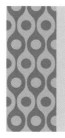

### ■ GRATITUDE LIST

From here throughout the rest of the program, write a list of at least five gratitudes daily.

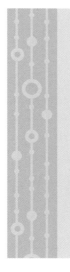

### Recipe: BROILED CAULIFLOWER WITH SEA SALT AND OLIVE OIL

This is one of my favorite healthy comfort food discoveries because it is a cinch to prepare, tastes like potatoes, but has only a fraction of the carbohydrates and calories. And it seems gourmet!

Take a cauliflower head and break apart into florets. Place in a bowl and drizzle with olive oil. Dust generously with sea salt. Mix it up. Place on a pan in the oven and broil until browned. Enjoy!

# DAY 5

## THINK YOUR WAY THIN

### Energy Flows Where the Mind Goes

**Y**ou have probably heard the saying, "You are what you eat," but let's take this a step further—what if you are what you *think?* Your mind is a powerful tool. The thoughts you think, both consciously and subconsciously, are the messages you send to yourself throughout the day and are vital to your life force, or lack thereof. If your mind is elsewhere, so is your energy. Energy flows where the mind goes. What are you feeding yourself mentally?

> "We can't solve problems using the same kind of thinking that created them."
>
> — ALBERT EINSTEIN

Noticing your thoughts is a good first step to understanding and being able to redirect how you create your view of yourself and your experiences. The more adept you become at observing your thoughts, the better you will be at directing them toward your desired outcome. Let me give you an example: When I am in a yoga pose, sometimes I notice myself wishing it were over or wanting to move on to the next thing. Then I recognize that my thought patterns are repetitive and habitual; in fact, I find myself running the same three thoughts over and over again in my mind. When I practice yoga, I get a chance to slow down long enough to witness my thoughts—and reframe them so that "This pose is hard" can be changed to "This is the feeling of my body getting stronger."

Along the same vein, telling yourself you're fat is not going to make you thinner any faster. These thoughts only defeat your purpose while you damage and terrorize yourself in the process—in fact, reinforcing what you don't want.

I recently read that worrying is like praying for what you don't want. Still, we are all prone to future-tripping, myself included. Just the other day I was feeling great when I started to imagine a "What if . . . ?" I was thinking up a scenario that never even happened, and then I started dialoguing with the person who had, in my imagination, wronged me. I was now having a fictional conversation based on an imaginary event, and I became completely unhinged. This is progress for me, because at least I was aware of it. I used to go up into my head and make up self-defeating stories without even realizing it! To the outside world, I was just driving along in my car, listening to the radio on my way to the market. But inside, I had created an emotional hurricane. Even though I knew I had invented it, my emotions were completely stirred. I went to a spinning class so I could burn the extra emotional energy—and I had boundless amounts at that point! This brings me to the conclusion that while emotions fuel my body, my mind rules my emotions.

Once you start to pay attention to your self-talk, be mindful of the thoughts you are reinforcing into your body. In fact, one of the best places where you can practice observing your thoughts is during exercise. Notice the voices in your head, both the ones that are trying to distract you and convince you that you are not good enough, as well as the encouraging voices. The more adept you become at directing your thoughts, the better you will be able to drive them toward your desired outcome. Until you can reframe the negative voices, the positive ones will remain obscured.

Today when you practice your Yogalosophy routine, notice what you are telling yourself. If there is anything that is not helpful, don't replace it at first. Own it, hang out with it. Know that this thought is yours. I really don't want you to remove or erase anything. What you have been using up until now has served you well. It got you right here, but it's time to try something different to see if it brings a different, better result. Once you have accepted your self-talk, you can start to reframe it by finding the positive spin.

The first step is to identify your self-defeating phrases. Then you can begin to reframe them.

Here are some examples:

- "I have a big butt" becomes "I am curvy and feminine."

- "I am exhausted and can't do this anymore" becomes "Breakthroughs come after breakdowns."

- "I'm dying" becomes "I can feel my body changing."

- "This is impossible" becomes "This is a challenge."

The beauty of yoga is the gift of slowing down enough to start to log those thoughts. Let's give them a place to live and evolve.

## ⊗ ACTION CHECKLIST

### INTENTION: *Go out of your mind!*

You are what you think. Pay attention to the words you say to yourself and the thoughts you think. Write a new script. Look in the mirror and say "I Love You." Do this daily. I know this sounds excruciating. That's what I first felt when I was given the assignment, but now I pass it along to you.

### PLAYLIST: *Changes*

This playlist was made with the intention of changing the mood of the music with each song. There is also a lot of spaciousness in some of the songs so that you can zone out.

"I Love Baby Cheesy," Banco de Gaia

"Scar Tissue," Red Hot Chili Peppers

"Bring on the Night," Police

"I Will Survive," Gloria Gaynor

"Goin' Out of My Head," Fatboy Slim

"Everyday Is a Winding Road," Sheryl Crow

"Je Danse Donc Je Suis," Brigette Bardot

"Push Upstairs," Underworld

"The Chain," Fleetwood Mac

"I Feel Love," Donna Summer

"I Confess," English Beat

"End of the Party," English Beat

### YOGALOSOPHY ROUTINE VARIATION

No yoga today! You will only do the toners, but will increase your reps (see next page). Enjoy the kinetic movement. Our thoughts are very rapid. Today we want to keep the movement rapid to mirror the mind.

### CARDIO OPTION

Do a thirty-minute cardio routine on an elliptical trainer or treadmill. Every two minutes, change it up by adding resistance, skipping, adding an incline, etc. The point is that you don't stay in the same movement and go on automatic pilot. Changing the movement will keep you alert and involved today. Get out of the head and into the legs.

DAY 5

# TONERS

See Yogalosophy Routine for photos (pages 10–24).

### CALF RAISES

Stand with your heels touching and your toes turned out at a forty-five-degree angle. If you need the wall or a chair for balance, feel free to use it. Elevate on to the balls of your feet. After three sets of ten, pulse the move for ten at the top.

### SQUATS

Stand tall with feet slightly wider than hip-width apart. Bring your hands on to your hips, and keep the weight even through the entire foot as you shift your hips back and lower into a squat. Squeeze as you press back to standing, squeezing slightly at the top of your full range of motion. Repeat three sets of ten. At the end of the last set, pulse down into mini-squats for ten.

### LUNGES

Step your left leg back. With the back knee slightly bent, hips tucked under and the right leg at a ninety-degree angle, lunge. Make sure that the knee it tracking directly over the center of the foot (over the third toe). Do three sets of ten. At the end of the last ten lunges, pulse down for ten. Repeat on other side.

### PLIÉ SQUATS

Step your feet wide apart, angling your toes out so that they are at the ten o'clock and two o'clock positions. Do not turn your feet out too much; you want the knees to track comfortably over the toes. Make sure that your back is straight and that you are not leaning the chest forward. Lower down into a plié squat and squeeze your inner thighs to draw yourself up to standing. Do thirty reps, then pulse for ten.

### EXTENDED LEG LIFTS

Come into a Downward Facing Dog or onto the hands and knees. Extend the right leg back behind you with a straight leg. Lower your leg to the floor and then, using your glutes, raise the leg back up. Repeat fifteen times with a flexed foot and fifteen with a pointed toe. Pulse for ten reps at the end. Repeat on other side.

## BENT-KNEE LEG LIFTS

Come onto your forearms and tilt your pelvis down, rounding your spine. Make sure you are not letting your back sway. Bend your knee at a ninety-degree angle and flex your foot so that the sole of the foot is aiming to the ceiling. Keep in mind that the knee should never drop lower than hip level. Pulse for forty. Switch sides.

## SIDE LEG LIFTS

Reach your right arm out to the side and support your body weight with your hand. Keeping the knee bent at a ninety-degree angle, lift it out to the side, then bring the right knee down to meet the left knee. Do thirty reps. Pulse for ten at the top. Repeat on other side.

## SUPERMAN

Lie flat on your stomach with arms outstretched to the sides, as if you are the letter T. Lift your chest, arms, and legs up, and then lower down. Repeat thirty reps and ten pulses. This move strengthens your back.

## PUSH-UPS

Come onto all fours, and either with straight legs or bent knees, lower your chest so that you are six inches above the floor. Hug your elbows into your ribs, close to your sides. Repeat three sets, pulse for ten.

## TRICEP PUSH-UPS

Sit down and place your hands on the floor behind you facing your heels. Place the feet on the floor and lift your hips. Aim your elbows back as you lower down and push up. Do twenty reps.

## PELVIC TUCKS

Lay down on your back with your knees bent, soles of your feet on the floor. Squeeze your glutes, as you press your hips up, and then lower them down. After thirty reps, pulse ten times at the top.

## CRISSCROSS ABS

Lie on your back with your feet on the floor. Cross your right ankle over your left knee and allow your right knee to open out to the right. Support your head with your left hand and hold the outside of the right knee. Twist your left elbow over to the right knee, engaging the obliques. Repeat thirty times and pulse for ten at the top. Switch sides.

## V-UPS

Begin in Bent-Knee Boat, balancing on tush. Lower the upper body until hovering six inches off the floor, at the same time extending the legs to hover six inches off the floor. On a strong exhale, draw your chest up and your knees into your chest, using your abdominals. Do four sets of ten.

## POSE OF THE DAY

### CHILD'S POSE

Kneel with your hips to your heels, arms extended straight, stretching as far away in front of you as possible, head resting on the floor. Feel your spine lengthening. This yoga pose is one of my favorites and will allow your mind to let go after all of the kinetic movement. Use this pose throughout the day to ground you if your mind goes into overdrive.

PHYSICAL BENEFITS: Stretches and tones hips, thighs, and ankles.

HEALING BENEFITS: Brings circulation to the face. Great for back and neck pain.

EMOTIONAL ASPECTS: Reduces stress, anxiety, and depression.

MODIFICATIONS: If you have difficulty bringing the hips to the heels, roll up a towel and place behind your knees.

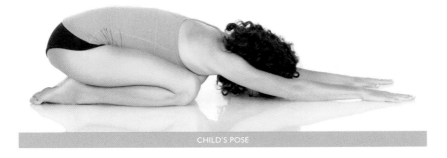

CHILD'S POSE

## EXTRA CREDIT: *Splurge on a journal.*

Today, you have an option to start keeping a daily journal (see below). Go to a stationary store or a boutique and pick out a journal with a cover design, colors, and paper texture that inspire you. I tend to favor a large black journal without lines. It feels like a blank canvas tht is wide open for my ideas. The key is to find a journal that inspires you to want to capture your thoughts, insights, and reflections it it. After all, your thoughts and feelings are valuable and deserve to be treated as such.

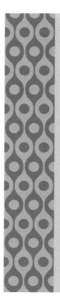

■ **START A JOURNAL**

Journaling is a very powerful way to reveal what you are saying to yourself, and how that self-talk is showing up in your body and your actions. Watch your mind and see where it is wandering.

What negative self-talk did you find yourself speaking today? Free-write about it. Where does it come from; what does it remind you of? Has it helped you in any way? What is the flip side, or the positive spin?

Write as much as you'd like, but spend at least ten minutes doing so.

Option: Do this daily for the remainder of the program.

■ **GRATITUDE LIST**

## *Recipe:* NUTS TO KEEP YOU FROM GOING NUTS

I love to snack, so I'm always looking for healthy solutions to feed my craving when I am on the go.

**2 cups raw nuts (use a mixture of your favorites. I go heavy on almonds, which are high in protein)**
**1 tablespoon olive oil**
**3 tablespoons furikake (an Asian mixture of sesame seeds, chopped nori, and other ingredients—you can usually purchase this in the Asian section of your grocery store.)**

Preheat oven to 350°F. Mix olive oil with the nuts to coat them. Evenly spread the nuts on a cookie sheet and bake until nicely browned, approximately 10 to 12 minutes. Remove nuts from oven and allow to cool slightly. Mix nuts together with furikake and store in an airtight container.

# DAY 6

## JUST BREATHE

### *Breath Is the Bridge from the Mind to the Body*

**B**reath is the key to life. It is the vehicle that carries the prana (or life-force energy) throughout your entire body. Breathing with intention calms you, giving you more presence as well as far more personal power. Even simple awareness of your breath, particularly the space between the inhale and the exhale (and vice versa), reconnects you with your center.

I once heard a great guideline for breathing that goes: Inhale. Exhale. Continue. Still, yoga breathing gets a lot of people confused. There are multiple techniques, and students regularly ask me if they are breathing correctly. Take my word for it: If you are still alive, you are doing it right. That said, in this chapter you'll find several breathing tips that will help you get the most out of each intentional breath.

But first, I'd like to share with you a bit about my own challenges with learning to really breathe. When I was a little girl, I skinned my knee. I wanted reassurance. So the

> *"I took a deep breath and listened to the old bray of my heart: I am, I am, I am."*
>
> — SYLVIA PLATH

memory of my dad screaming, "BREATHE!" at me was enough to send me into a lifelong rebellion against the very thing that keeps me alive. To this day, I often find myself holding my breath. When I have an important meeting, or I'm being interviewed on the air, or even when I am teaching, I have to remind myself to breathe. Breathing techniqus are used consciously as a centering force in everything from anxiety and sleep-disorder programs to birthing and athletics.

As I mentioned earlier, the breath builds the bridge from the mind to the body. We often carry pent-up emotions, and when you hold your breath, it gives you an illusion of control. But it takes energy to hold on to tension—energy that could be directed at something more useful and positive. I find that when I breathe my emotions are freed. If you practice breathing and let go of your restraints and allow those feelings and emotions to flow out through each breath, you will be amazed at how much more energy and life force you have. As you concentrate on breathing, your mental chatter will disperse, and you'll experience more presence of mind, clarity, and focus. In short, it feels amazing!

## YOGA BREATHING TIP #1: *Go with the Flow*

Generally in yoga, we connect breath with movement. In fact, the Sanskrit word *vinyasa,* which you hear in many yoga classes, means linking the breath with body movement. The inhalation is generally taken when we expand the body. The exhalation occurs when we contract. When you expand the lungs by leaning back into an arch, it feels natural to take in as much breath as possible, and when folding in to a forward bend or a contraction, it makes sense to expel the air.

## YOGA BREATHING TIP# 2: *Nose Your Way Through*

Breathe in and out of the nose. The mouth is generally kept closed during a yoga practice. Breathing through your nose heats your body while increasing your lung capacity. The jaw should be relaxed and the throat should be slightly constricted, which will create a hollow sound or an "ocean breath," also called *ujjayi* (ooh-JAI-ee) or "victory breath."

## YOGA BREATHING TIP #3: *Belly Up!*

This is like a baby's breath where the belly fills completely on the inhale and deflates on the exhale. Begin by expanding the belly, then the ribs, and finally the chest. Release them down as you exhale fully through the nose. This will also help tone the abdominal muscles.

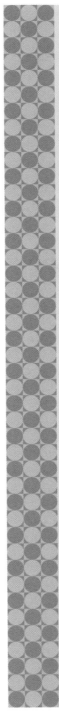

## ✳ ACTION CHECKLIST

**INTENTION:** *Watch the movie.*

If you are like me, you may have a very active mind that projects stories and images all day long. Become aware of the home movies you are projecting on to the screen of your mind. As you notice your latest personal blockbuster playing in the background of your yoga practice and during your day, try to bring your awareness back to your breath.

In fact, while you're at it, notice how many times during the day you find yourself holding your breath! It's okay to have distractions, but try to remember to take a long inhale and exhale. Every time you find yourself distracted—checking your cell phone or rushing—make it a reminder to reconnect with the breath. This way your habitual patterns become your reminder.

**PLAYLIST:** *Breathe*

This playlist will remind you to breathe, either through words, or through the spacious rhythmic songs:

"Breathe Me," Sia

"Breathe In," Frou Frou

"Barely Breathing," Duncan Sheik

"The Air That I Breathe," The Hollies

"Lean On Me," Aural Encounter

"My Friend," Groove Armada

"Lebanese Blonde," Thievery Corporation

"At The River," Groove Armada

"Angels," Wax Poetic

"Make Love," Daft Punk

"All I Need," Air

"Another Woman," Moby

"Astral Weeks," Van Morrison

"Heart Sutra Soulshine," Wah!

**YOGALOSOPHY ROUTINE VARIATION**

Hold each posture for three to five breaths, primarily focusing on the ujjayi yoga breathing.

**CARDIO OPTION**

Today, instead of a cardio routine, add the breathing exercises in this chapter. Begin with three rounds of Breath of Fire, and end with three rounds of Alternate Nostril Breathing. Use ujjayi breathing throughout your practice, and take deep breaths throughout the day. In fact, one of the greatest benefits of cardiovascular work is connection to the breath. If you do not want to do the techniques described here, go on a run to access breathing.

DAY 6

# BREATHING

As a child, I could always hear my father practicing yoga before I could see him. I knew he was practicing before I even came downstairs because it sounded like Darth Vadar from Star Wars. A constriction at the back of the throat creates the hollow sound. It is a deep, full-belly breath that is done with a closed mouth. It is sometimes referred to as Ocean Breath, because it sounds like the rhythm of the ocean.

- Find a comfortable seated position.

- Focus on the breath moving in and out of your nose.

- Place your hands on your belly and allow the breath to fill your belly and your belly to expand into your hand on each inhale. Have you ever noticed that when a baby breathes, its entire body expands on the inhale, as if it's breathing through its entire torso? That's the result you want. On the exhale, the belly will draw inward naturally.

- Now try this. On the next exhale, let out a soundless "HAAA," as if you were to whisper "HAAA." Repeat this a few times.

- Next do the same thing, but close your mouth, imagining that you are exhaling the "HAAA" whisper with a closed mouth.

This is Ujjayi breathing, or Ocean Breath. You can continue to practice, incorporating this type of breathing into your yoga practice. Don't be concerned if you feel awkward at first; it will come with repetition.

This heating exercise, which is done with your mouth closed, is a vigorous fast-paced breath from your navel, primarily using force to exhale out, while taking tiny sips of air in, but the emphasis is on the contraction of the abs as you force the air out through your nose. When you exhale, the breath is thrown out with such force that you naturally have to take a breath in so don't focus on the inhale. This is a purification breath, and you will feel your abdominals working. Be patient; this technique takes some coordination and practice.

- Sit tall in a comfortable position.

- Take three slow Ujjayi breaths to prepare.

- Inhale the fourth time, and with force, pull your belly in as you exhale out your nose. Move your abdominal sheath in and out by putting the attention about two inches behind the belly button. Do not pause between the breaths. Keep pulling your naval in to force the breath out. You will naturally take small sips of air in.

- Increase your speed, keeping the breath in your belly.

- Maintain the breathing for one minute.

Once you have finished, hold the breath on the last inhale and then let out an exhale.

You may feel lightheaded. That is common. If you need to take breaks or feel out of control at any time, stop and rest in Child's Pose. You can work up to three minutes with this technique.

## ALTERNATE NOSTRIL BREATHING

This cooling breath-work creates balance between the logical and creative parts of your brain. This is the optimal way to calm the nervous system.

- Sit cross-legged. Using your right hand, place your thumb on your right nostril and your ring finger on your left nostril. Rest your index and middle finger on the bridge of your nose. Then do the following steps. Repeat three times to complete three rounds of alternate nostril breathing.

- Slowly inhale through the left nostril, closing the right with the thumb while counting to four.

- Now hold the breath, closing both nostrils, and count to sixteen.

- Exhale through the right nostril, closing the left with the ring and little finger while counting to eight.

- Inhale through the right nostril, keeping the left closed with the ring and little finger, for a count of four.

- Hold the breath, closing both nostrils for a count of sixteen.

- Exhale through the left nostril, keeping the right closed with the thumb.

Breath is such an amazing tool. It is your body's natural, built-in coolant and heating system. When you need to warm up, simply closing the mouth keeps the heat inside your body. Think of your belly as a furnace, and the breath is fanning that fire in your belly. When you need to cool down, try opening the mouth as you exhale. Begin to bring more mindfulness to your breathing and notice your breathing patterns. You can always take a deep breath to press the reset button.

## POSE OF THE DAY

### SIDE PLANK

It takes practice to find balance, but one of the keys is connecting to the consistent rhythm of your breath. The idea for balance is to connect with something consistent. If you think of breathing as the natural rhythm of your personal ocean, you will understand how this is something you can (and do!) rely on.

Begin in Plank pose, with feet together.

Move your right hand directly below your face and at the center of the mat.

Rock your body to the right side, stacking the feet on top of each other as you balance on your right hand and the outside edge of the right foot. Or keep the feet hip width apart and rock onto the sides of both feet for added balance. Flex your feet and make sure the underside of the waist lifts upwards so that your top hip is pressing toward the ceiling.

Keep your head, shoulders, hips, and heels in one line. You may need to scoop your tailbone under, open the chest to the sky, and draw the top hip forward.

Press your right palm into the floor so that you are rebounding off of the mat. Be aware that you are not hyperextending or locking your elbow. Repeat on opposite side.

PHYSICAL BENEFITS: Strengthens and tones arms, belly, legs, and obliques.

HEALING BENEFITS: Brings focus to a scattered mind.

EMOTIONAL ASPECTS: Calms the spirit. Centers the body.

MODIFICATIONS: Bring bottom knee to floor for support. For more of a challenge, raise the top leg.

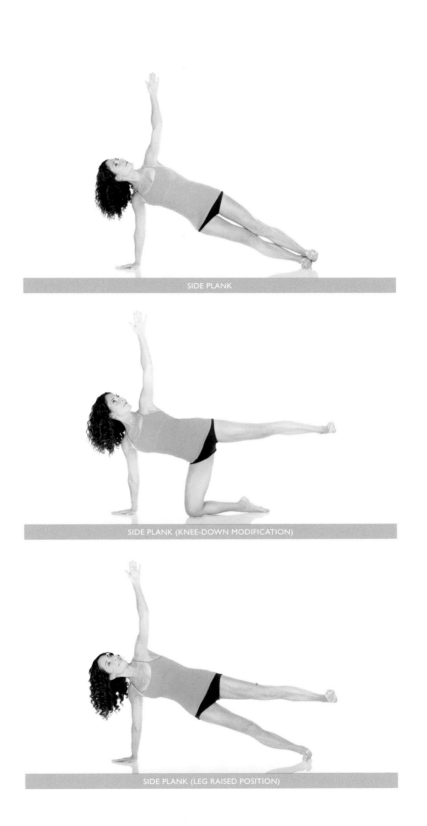

SIDE PLANK

SIDE PLANK (KNEE-DOWN MODIFICATION)

SIDE PLANK (LEG RAISED POSITION)

## EXTRA CREDIT: *Make space for you.*

Get a manicure or a shoulder massage. This will loosen you up and help create space to breathe more openly.

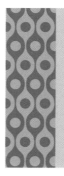

■ **JOURNAL**

When did you find yourself holding your breath today? What was coming up for you, and how did you catch yourself? How did it feel to take a deep breath in that moment?

■ **GRATITUDE LIST**

## ℛecipe: KALE SALAD WITH MISO DRESSING

1 head kale, destemmed and chopped
1 tablespoon olive oil
¼ cup pine nuts
½ cup halved cherry tomatoes
¼ cup thinly sliced fennel

Place kale in large salad bowl. Drizzle with olive oil and dash of salt. Massage kale with your hands for a few minutes. This makes it more digestable. Add tomatoes, fennel, and pine nuts and toss with dressing.

### MISO DRESSING:

1 diced shallot
1 tablespoon Dijon mustard
1 tablespoon mellow white miso
¼ cup unsweetened, rice vinegar
4 drops stevia extract
3 tablespoons of extra-virgin olive oil

Blend in a blender cup or shake well to mix.

# DAY 7

## EMOTION: PUT YOUR ENERGY IN MOTION
### *Feel Your Way Through*

E motions are our primary motivating force in life. Pretty much everything we aspire to do, from career goals to the friends and partners we choose, are driven by our emotions. What's more, I believe our emotional roots—and the habits that form with them—begin in the womb and evolve through the teachings of our parents as we grow up. For that reason, I consider our parents the foundation of our emotional motivations.

Taking that notion of parental influence a step further, my theory is that diet is the mother of the body, and exercise is the father. Food is the support and nurturing that sustains me and gives me nourishment and the grounding I need in order to give life to all of my dreams. Exercise stretches and pushes me past my limitations, inspires me to move forward, and challenges me to develop strength and independence.

Of course many of us have had or still have complicated relationships with our actual parents, and likewise we tend to develop complicated relationships with food and exercise. Regardless, for better or worse

> *"It is my fervent hope that my whole life on this earth will ever be tears and laughter."*
>
> — KAHLIL GIBRAN

our foundation is made up of these relationships—mother/food, father/exercise—so it's essential that we learn how to leverage and evolve the best of our familial experiences, leave what no longer works behind, and become our own best parent.

I have learned to self-parent through trial and error, taking the best of what each parent has given me. I'll tell you more about my mom tomorrow, but today let me tell you about my dad, Lloyd Ingber. As a child, I had a tumultuous relationship with him. He was very young when he became a father; I came along when he was in his early twenties, just as he was getting to know himself and exploring the '70s cultural revolution. He used to joke that we grew up together, which isn't far from the truth. When I was six or seven years old, my father began to practice yoga and became an Iyengar master, even as he maintained a successful career as an attorney. Our family would even go to a weekly group class together.

My parents had plans to start a side business called "PEP: Productivity Enhancement Program," which they dreamed would bring yoga into offices so that instead of a coffee break, there would be a yoga break. Although PEP never happened, my father cultivated his yoga practice in the entry hall of our Bel Air home. On any given day you'd walk downstairs and hear *Happy Days* blaring in the background, while Dad was doing his Darth Vader breathing, in some contortionist pose, usually with his leg behind his head. As effortless as his yogic poise seemed, he could just as easily unravel and lash out with his temper. That's why I have no illusions about yoga eliminating all negativity; sometimes when we practice, we feel our emotions, both positive and negative, even more . . . although without yoga, I am sure it could be worse. Possibly, because of my father, my personal work has been to observe my emotions and use them toward positive actions. I am not always successful. Ask my bank teller.

I learned to emulate my dad. My father was a businessman out in the world, but a yogi at home. In an effort to get close to him, I would contort myself for his praise; but more than that, I think it was a desire to experience what he was experiencing. If I could be in a pose like the one he was in, if I could read the books he read, then maybe I could understand him better. For a long time, I didn't. We fought endlessly, for years.

He died of cancer when he was sixty years old. I grieved in part for what I did not get from my dad. Then, one day, I was in Downward Facing Dog for the first time after he died, and I realized that he had passed something on to me that connected me to an entire lineage. It took me until he was gone to really understand what he gave me: the gift of yoga, the presence and freedom to be found in movement—this was my most valuable inheritance. My father's daily practice was constant throughout his sixty years. His tenacity to overcome all obstacles was contagious, and I adopted these qualities as my own. And now I get to take the best of what he gave me and pass that along to others—including you.

Ultimately, my relationship with my dad taught me that emotions are just fuel, something to be used in my life rather than something that controls my life. I'm a very emotional person, so this understanding didn't come easily to me. Here's what I mean: When I was a kid, I was so afraid of The Wicked Witch that Mom cut out all of the scary pictures from my storybooks. There were just a bunch of empty holes where the witch used to be. She meant well, but one of the results was that I didn't learn to manage my feelings. So with no coping mechanisms in place a little later in life, I became afraid that if I allowed myself to feel sad or fearful, I would fall into a bottomless pit.

As I got older and got more seriously into yoga and exercise, I learned that just breathing and moving my body shifts things. I began to understand that having emotions doesn't mean that I *am* my emotions. When I am moving my body, feelings come up and energy literally moves! I may be sad, but if I I just exercise, I usually feel a lot better afterward.

I also learned that emotions find a way to be expressed through the body in one way or another, consciously or unconsciously. For example, I once had a verbally abusive boss who made my work life hell. I couldn't hide the stress I was under, and my back gave out completely—one morning I woke up and couldn't even roll over. Another time I was having trouble moving on from a breakup with a boyfriend, and I developed a knee injury, a perfect metaphor for not being able to move forward. Time and again, my emotions have expressed themselves through my physical being.

It is not always appropriate to yell back at a boss or possible to eliminate fears of your proverbial Wicked Witch, just as it's not possible to fix our parents or make someone love us, I know. But I do know that you can always funnel what you are feeling through your body and into your exercise. You don't have to feel perfect in order to move—and it will alleviate some of your body's built-up emotion. A great example is a client who came to work out with me on a day when she was really mad about some career issues. When I started asking her questions about it, she became so mad she didn't even realize she was working out. I had never seen her run faster! Her anger had transformed her into a superhero. Emotions are powerful and can fuel us.

Over the years, I have come to consider these teachings my emotional roots. Today we'll look at using our emotional roots as a way to keep motivated. Whatever you are feeling right now is a great starting point.

## ✿ ACTION CHECKLIST

**INTENTION:** *Feel your way through.*

Emotions, like water, are fluid. Today, get into the flow. For starters, add the below Flow sequence between your poses in your Yogalosophy workout today. Additionally, drink more water. When you find yourself emotionally charged, water can flush it out.

**PLAYLIST:** *Energy In Motion*

When I was a spinning instructor, I learned that different types of music evoke different emotions. This playlist may make you feel angry, sad, or passionate. Use the emotional energy to drive you through.

"Harvey and the Old Ones," Banco
  de Gaia

"Paid in Full," Erik B. and Rakim

"Love Me With a Feeling," Bette Midler

"All Apologies," Nirvana

"Break On Through," The Doors

"Warning Sign," Coldplay

"No More Drama," Mary J. Blige

"Feeling for You," Cassius

"You Make Me Feel," Sylvester

"Feeling Alright," Joe Cocker

"Make Me Wanna Holla," Me'shell
  Ndegeocello

**YOGALOSOPHY ROUTINE VARIATION**

Add Sun Salutations. Either weave this sequence between each set of the Y28 poses and toners to make the routine more fluid, or begin with ten to fifteen Sun Salutations before the routine. The Sun Salutation also incorporates the breathing we have begun to access, connecting movement with breath, which will flood your body with otherwise blocked emotion.

**CARDIO OPTION**

Add water! Go for a twenty-minute swim. Take a bath.

DAY 7

# POSES OF THE DAY

## Sun Salutation/Flow Sequence

PHYSICAL BENEFITS: Total body workout: tones arms, abs, legs. Stretches entire back and front of the body. Engages breath.

HEALING BENEFITS: Tones the digestive system, regulates menstrual cycle, ventilates lungs, and oxygenates blood.

EMOTIONAL ASPECTS: Lifts the spirits, calms the mind, and increases energy.

MODIFICATIONS: Option A: Bring knees to the floor for Plank. Option B: Keep the thighs on the floor for Upward Facing Dog. Option C: Replace Downward Facing Dog with Child's Pose. If none of these work, try just breathing and moving.

### MOUNTAIN POSE

Mountain pose is a foundational pose, which is why we keep returning to it. It is essentially "home base" in your practice. You will return to it again and again. It can be found within all of the Hatha yoga poses, and it is a guideline to assess proper alignment. Begin with feet parallel and touching. Lift your kneecaps by firming the thighs and tuck the tailbone just slightly as you draw your navel in and up while extending out of the waist. Draw your shoulders back and down, arms loose at your sides, palms facing out. Lengthen through the crown of your head.

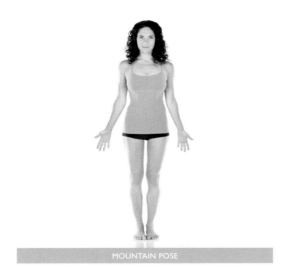

MOUNTAIN POSE

## FORWARD BEND

From Mountain, swan dive down with a flat back, arms sweeping out into a forward bend. Take five breaths here. Place your fingertips on the floor and extend your spine before moving into Plank.

## PLANK

Place your palms on the mat below your shoulders. Step the feet back and together, while keeping your body in a strong, straight line by engaging your stabilizing and abdominal muscles. Imagine the Mountain pose within this Plank.

## LOW PLANK

Lower your body down from Plank, keeping the elbows close to the sides of your body. Stop when your shoulders and elbows are aligned. Hover as you look straight ahead.

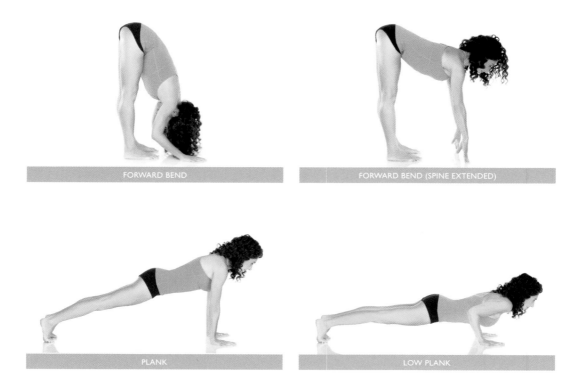

FORWARD BEND

FORWARD BEND (SPINE EXTENDED)

PLANK

LOW PLANK

## UPWARD FACING DOG

Turn the tops of your feet to the floor and press them into the mat as you press the palms into the floor. On the inhale, look up and lift your chest up until your arms are straight, allowing your upper thighs and knees to lift off of the floor. Lower down and transition to Downward Facing Dog.

## DOWNWARD FACING DOG

Turn the balls of your feet under and, on the exhale, push away from the floor as you raise your hips up to an inverted "V" position. Press evenly through your entire palm. Relax your head and neck and make sure your spine is straight. Feel free to bend your knees if your hamstrings are tight. Allow your heels to sink toward the floor. Breathe.

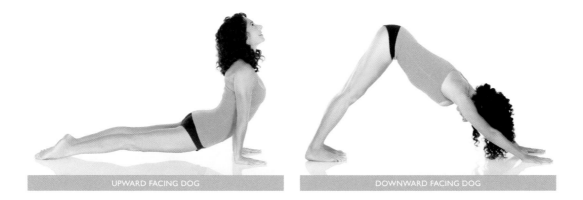

UPWARD FACING DOG         DOWNWARD FACING DOG

## EXTRA CREDIT: *Tap into your heart.*

Be present with your feelings and allow them to fuel you.

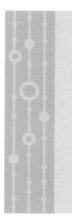

■ **JOURNAL**

If you choose, you may continue to journal each day. There will be occasional questions to provoke you. Journaling is one of the most helpful ways to express what you really feel.

■ **GRATITUDE LIST**

■ **BREATHING EXERCISE**

From here on out, try to incorporate one or more of the breathing exercises from Day 6 (pages 78–80) into your routine. Breathing with intention will not only help ground you, it will also improve the flow of life-force energy through your body as you move throughout each day.

## *Recipe:* INFUSED WATER

**OPTION 1:** Slice cucumbers, oranges, and lemon and place in a pitcher. Add filtered water and chill.

**OPTION 2:** To spruce up your water, mix four ounces of unsweetened cranberry juice with six ounces of sparkling water. Add a touch of stevia, the natural, no-calorie sweetener, to taste. Yummy and refreshing.

# DAY 8

## NURTURE YOURSELF

*Doing Nothing Is Something*

ontinuing with yesterday's topic of emotional roots, I believe that as father energy inspires, mother energy supports. One of the things I hear most often from my students is that I have a nurturing quality. I feel that my purpose is to hold space while the student finds his or her way through what can sometimes be a challenging physical practice. I feel honored when I play the witness and simply contain the experience. The balance between helping to guide and providing the space for the process, rather than doing it for the other person, is what I consider a nurturing quality. I am sure I picked this up from my mom.

> *"By letting it go, it all gets done. The world is won by those who let it go."*
>
> — LAO TZU

My mother was born in a displaced person's camp in Germany. After World War II, when she was three, she came to the United States by boat with my uncle and grandparents. As a little girl in a new land, my mom taught her own parents how to speak English. She would go to school and come home with the latest lessons. At age twenty, she was virtually a child when she had me. My brother Dave was born when she was twenty-one.

My brother and I were raised with loving patience and lots of comedy; Mom was always keeping us entertained with Rolling Stones impressions. While cooking five-course macrobiotic meals for our family, she would imitate Mick Jagger, transforming a wooden spoon into a microphone. She turned me on to Steve Martin and Albert Brooks on *Saturday Night Live,* and cultivated the irreverence and humor that would color my entire childhood. Mom was a natural nurturer and teacher. I definitely got my teaching abilities and sense of humor from her.

She had a tendency, however, to take care of others first, and then lick the serving bowls clean for her own dinner. I kept the nurture, but ultimately had to learn to feed myself first.

Our society trains us to become achievers, but there is such value in providing the support for all of your dreams to come true. Not all of you had a mom that gave you puppet shows at bedtime or who even had the time to cook for you. There are all sorts of parents out there, and as an adult, you must fill in the blanks for yourself. You must create for yourself a space that contains and supports you. You must self-nurture.

Nurture is the foundation of all that you will accomplish. I run around a lot, and find that establishing a sense of home base is extra challenging. Having spent a lot of my life being hypercritical, forcing my body, and depriving myself, I had actually convinced myself that this type of self-abuse was what motivation looked like. I actually thought that was the key to my accomplishments. It turns out that when I remove that slave-driving voice and replace it with healthy choices and loving self-talk that helps me to reason out my less nurturing decisions, my body falls into place effortlessly, and I actually begin to feel the loving relationship with myself that I need. My food cravings subside because I am getting the right kind of mothering, and it isn't through ice cream—although I do sample salty dark chocolate on a fairly regular basis.

If you're like my mom and me, you tend to feed others first. You put everyone before yourself. Your spouse, children, parents, friends, your boss, even your pet may get more attention and care than you give to yourself. However, even if it seems there is not enough time in the day to meet all of the needs of others and provide support for yourself, you must find a way to make time and prioritize yourself as the most important being to nurture. We learn from and teach by example. The best way to nurture is to be an example of self-nurturing. When your loved ones see you feeding them and not caring for yourself, it teaches them that nurturing is depleting, when it is the opposite! Be the example.

## ✺ ACTION CHECKLIST

**INTENTION:** *Be receptive.*

In the ancient mysticism of Kabbalah, they say that the ultimate act of giving is to receive. This makes sense to me, in that when I have felt "received" in my life it has always made me feel so good. In order to make the universe feel good, receive the bounty of its gifts today. That can mean receiving others in your arms through hugs, or receiving compliments graciously. Even a criticism from another may have the seed of a gift within it. Imagine that everything occurring today is a gift for you to receive.

### PLAYLIST

Choose your own playlist today. Use music to help you flow through your practice. Notice that when you play music and evoke different emotions, it actually drives your body.

### YOGALOSOPHY ROUTINE VARIATION

Sometimes it feels like we carry the world on our shoulders. By opening up the shoulders we also free our arms, which are extensions of our heart. We hold our loved ones in our arms, and we want to be able to provide that love and nurturing unhindered. In addition to the Yogalosophy routine, add the three shoulder-opening stretches shown on the following pages.

### CARDIO OPTION

No cardio today. Sweat it out at a steam bath or sauna. Or create an at-home spa: replenish yourself with a mineral bath, Jacuzzi, or long shower.

DAY 8

# POSES OF THE DAY

## Rabbit, Dolphin, Seated Shoulder Stretch

### RABBIT

Begin in Child's Pose. Rest your head on the floor, your torso on your thighs, your arms down by your side. Press your forehead on your knees and reach to hold on to the base of your feet. Inhale and on the exhalation slowly lift your hips, keeping your forehead close to your knees and the crown of the head on the floor. Contract your abs and hold the pose for two to three breaths and relax. Lower down. Rest.

> PHYSICAL BENEFITS: Aligns and stretches spine. Good for head, neck, and spine.
>
> HEALING BENEFITS: Massages thyroid. Improves posture.
>
> EMOTIONAL ASPECTS: Helps relieve insomnia and mild depression.
>
> MODIFICATIONS: Avoid putting too much pressure on the head and neck.

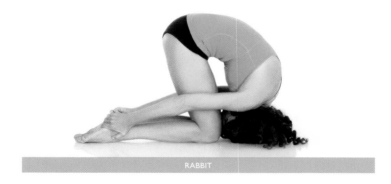

RABBIT

## DOLPHIN

Start on your hands and knees, with the knees directly below your hips. Place your forearms on the floor. Align your wrists and elbows. Curl your toes under and exhale as you raise your knees off of the floor, straightening your legs. Lift the sit bones toward the ceiling. Allow the heels to sink as the legs straighten. Actively press the forearms into the floor, as if you are rebounding off of the mat. Hang your head between the shoulders, allowing the traction to create a deep shoulder stretch. Keep your knees bent if your back is rounding. Lengthen your tailbone away from your pelvis as you extend your sternum toward the floor. Breathe five deep breaths. Bend your knees and come back to Child's Pose. Rest.

PHYSICAL BENEFITS: Strengthens upper back. Stretches shoulders, hamstrings, calves.

HEALING BENEFITS: Improves digestion. Relieves headaches, insomnia, back pain. Also therapeutic for high blood pressure.

EMOTIONAL ASPECTS: Relieves stress and mild depression.

MODIFICATIONS: Place your hands on a wall. Step your legs back, lengthen your torso, and allow the chest and shoulders to open. Or if hamstrings are tight, bend the knees.

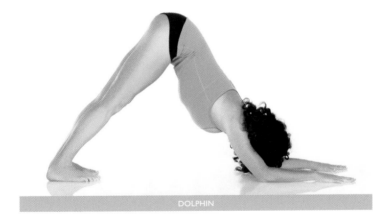

DOLPHIN

## SEATED SHOULDER STRETCH

Come into a kneeling position. As you sit up straight, extend your right arm straight up over your head on an inhale, bend the elbow, and touch your mid-back. Reach the left arm up and over to hold the right elbow for a gentle shoulder stretch. If you find this easy, reach the left arm behind you, bending the elbow and reach for the right hand, clasping the hands behind your back. Continue to sit up straight, extending your sternum toward the ceiling. You can lean your head back until it is in alignment with your spine. Breathe five times and then switch sides.

PHYSICAL BENEFITS: Opens the shoulders in preparation for Bridge (see page 108).

HEALING BENEFITS: Relieves tension in shoulders and strain in neck.

EMOTIONAL ASPECTS: Opens the heart.

MODIFICATIONS: Use a strap instead of clasping the hands. Or reach for elbow up and overhead.

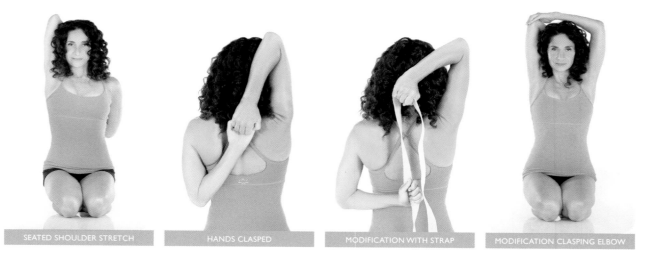

SEATED SHOULDER STRETCH     HANDS CLASPED     MODIFICATION WITH STRAP     MODIFICATION CLASPING ELBOW

## EXTRA CREDIT: *Receive love.*

Find a childhood photo of yourself and reconnect with that innocence. What love would you give that little kid? There is a part of me that is untouched from when I was a kid. Make a connection to that place within you. Give and receive hugs today.

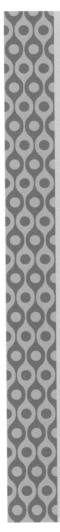

■ **JOURNAL**

Write a letter to the little child part of yourself from the future, with an assurance that everything is okay. Make sure to tell that little child how much you love her or him and that you are there and always will be.

■ **GRATITUDE LIST**

■ **BREATHING EXERCISE**

■ **DIET MODIFICATION:** *Week 2*

Congratulations on making a major shift in your diet last week. For week two, you can step it up a notch. This week includes a one-day OPTIONAL detox on Day 11. So in preparation, begin to add an extra liter of water to your diet each day. You should also choose to eat a large, healthy veggie-only salad for lunch for the next three days. This will prepare your body for a twenty-four-hour detox.

See page 122 for your cleanse guidelines.

Remember to listen to your body—and that this challenge is just an option. If you choose not to take the challenge, adding the extra liter of water and large helping of veggies should leave you feeling lighter anyway!

To recap:

- Add a liter of water (you are up to three).
- Replace one snack with green juice.
- Eat a large salad for lunch.
- Take the Detox Challenge on Day 11.

# Recipe: MANDY'S EARTH MAMA VEGAN STEW

I am not as active in the kitchen as I am in other areas, so one trick I learned was to toss everything in to a pot and make a soup or a stew! You can put in all sorts of veggies and legumes to make a large soup. You can feed a lot of people with it, and it lasts for days!

**2 cubes veggie bullion**
**1 32-ounce box of vegetable broth**
**½ cup legumes of choice (brown lentils, black beans, navy beans, adzuki beans)**
**2 carrots**
**3 celery stalks**
**½ onion**
**1 16-ounce can of tomato sauce**
**8 to 10 quartered small red potatoes**
**1 chopped medium leek**
**1 cup broccoli florets**
**5 to 8 chopped leaves of kale**
**1 thinly sliced scallion**
**2 tablespoons olive oil**
**2 cloves garlic**
**Spices: ½ teaspoon each of: garlic powder, paprika, sea salt, dried basil, oregano; ¼ teaspoon cumin**

Combine the garlic powder, paprika, salt, basil, oregano, and cumin in a small bowl. Heat oil in a large soup pot over medium to high heat and add garlic, onion, celery, carrot, potato, leek, broccoli, scallion, and kale. Stir in the seasonings and cook until onions are translucent and tender, stirring constantly.

Add the vegetable broth, tomato sauce, lentils, and veggie bullion cubes. Bring to a boil on high heat and then reduce to a low heat and simmer. Place the lid on, askew. Simmer for fifty minutes, or until lentils are cooked.

Add spices or water as needed to taste.

# DAY 9

## ACT AS IF

### *You Are the Star of Your Own Movie*

**H**ave you ever heard the self-help phrase "Fake it till you make it?" It's a notion that suggests that repeatedly acting out what you envision ultimately makes it real. When I first heard the phrase, I cringed, because I pride myself on being authentic. I didn't want to be "fake," and I didn't want to pretend that I was "making it" (whatever that means). Although the saying felt threatening at first, I've had firsthand experience with the value of acting your way into correct thinking and behaving the way you would if you felt like your best self.

> *"An ounce of behavior is worth a pound of words."*
>
> — SANFORD MEISNER

Let's look at it another way: Some actors act from the outside in, using costume or physical stance to access the inner life of a character. I love that when you see a show at the theater it's called a play. We are all just playing. An actor has an intention to project what he or she wants, and an emotional backstory that's driving that desire. There are actions that the character takes, and relationships or circumstances that evoke emotions, which drive the story. Then the actor has to be in the present moment, and be in relationship to the environment on the stage in order to create the reality of the character. Your life is a lot like this. So is your workout.

There is wisdom that can be gained from "acting as if," starting with behaving like you would if you were someone else. I have often asked myself, "What would a thin person eat?" and made food choices accordingly. A thin person does not need to be on a diet, so would not choose to drink diet soda. A thin person does not eat unconsciously either, but eats to fuel the body. We can use "acting" to motivate new behaviors.

Here's an example of how "acting as if" has helped me: Once a hummingbird flew into the house that I was house-sitting. I was the only person there and the bird was stuck very high up above a windowsill and did not seem to be able to find its way out. The little guy was very scared and there was no one to help but me. I called a friend. He was not available to come by, but he calmed me down enough for me to realize that I was going to have to go ahead and cup the bird in my hands, take it outside, and set it free. I was so freaked out by the frantic little bird, I didn't know how exactly to approach picking it up and wrapping my hands around it. My solution was to imagine what my nine-year-old friend, Deni, would do. She was a nature girl. All animals and insects loved her, and she loved them. I decided to act like I was Deni, and openly approached the bird, as she would have. I pretended and embodied her energy and what do you know—it worked! I got the little creature out of the house and held that delicate power in my hands before I set it free. What an amazing feeling!

This "acting as if" can also work in the negative. In kindergarten, I started playing a game on the playground before class with two male friends. One of the boys was on my side and the other boy would chase us; we were afraid of him in the playacting game. What started as a game became all too real, as we started to really not like the boy we were running away from. I took note of this, even as a little girl. "Hadn't this all started in the imagination?"

How you act is how you will feel, and the way you feel will bring about the behavior that will create the outcome. So why not act as if you can do anything! Today, as you work out, pretend you are a superhero, fitness instructor, your favorite actor, or a rock star!

## ✗ ACTION CHECKLIST

**INTENTION:** *Take center stage.*

Be a rock star. Are you Mick Jagger? Rihanna? Madonna? Be bold. Be as celebratory and big as you possibly can. As you go through your day, think of yourself as that character. How would they behave or handle the situation at hand. Enjoy your antics and see yourself as a performer on a stage. Have fun with it.

**PLAYLIST:** *Mandy's Party Playlist, circa 1988*

I made this mix for my twentieth birthday party and brought it back into my spinning classes when I was thirty. Now, into my forties, I am giving it to you. A good mix is always a good mix.

"Brick House," Commodores

"Super Freak," Rick James

"Goin' Back to Cali," LL Cool J

"Nasty Girl," Vanity 6

"Evil Ways," Santana

"Higher Love," Steve Winwood

"Kiss," Prince

"ABC," Jackson 5

"Love the One You're With," Crosby, Stills, Nash & Young

"The Joker," Steve Miller Band

"You Can Leave Your Hat On," Joe Cocker

"Let's Get It On," Marvin Gaye

**YOGALOSOPHY ROUTINE VARIATION**

Invite people over and have a yoga party. Have each person bring a favorite childhood treat. Do the standard Yogalosophy routine together and have fun. Then enjoy your well-earned treats. Remember: If you are preparing for the detox challenge on Day 11, a little sweetness goes a long way.

**CARDIO OPTION**

Dance Party. Have each of your friends bring a favorite song. If you have six people, you will have a thirty-minute cardio dance party. Trade off being in the center of the circle. Have fun and dance your ass off!

DAY 9

# POSE OF THE DAY

## ROCK STAR

Begin in Downward Facing Dog. Rotate your body to the right side, and place your weight on the outer edge of the right foot. Drop the ball of your left foot to the outside of the right knee as you press into the floor. Open your chest to the sky as you sweep your left arm back alongside your left ear and arch your body as you look up and back. Carefully bring your arm back up and over and bring your leg up behind you in Three-legged Dog. Then place the foot back to Downward Facing Dog and switch sides.

PHYSICAL BENEFITS: Strengthens shoulders, opens the chest. Stretches the entire front of the body.

HEALING BENEFITS: Tones the kidneys and adrenals.

EMOTIONAL ASPECTS: Lifts the spirits. Boosts energy.

MODIFICATIONS: If you are not used to the pose, do a modified backbend, like Bridge or Cat/Cow.

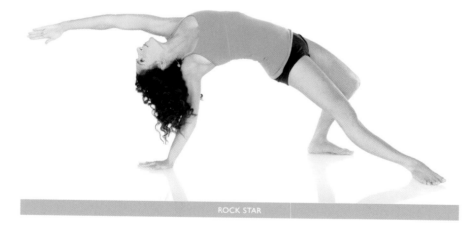

ROCK STAR

## EXTRA CREDIT: *Don't just work out, play out!*

Be bold today and really own your space. Dress up in your best gear, or wear a costume to your workout. Sometimes changing your look can be motivating. Extra credit if you do your workout in character.

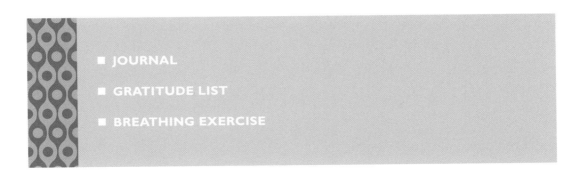

- JOURNAL
- GRATITUDE LIST
- BREATHING EXERCISE

# Recipe: MANDY'S FAVORITE MACROBIOTIC APPLE CRISP

This is a healthy but sweet one! When I was a child on a macrobiotic diet, my family put me in charge of dessert. When you eliminate sugar from your diet, your taste buds become much more receptive. This will taste amazingly yummy now that you have been off sugar for a week! In addition to your apple crisp, make sure to include a large all-vegetable salad for lunch to balance out your party indulgence.

**2 lbs. sliced apples**
**pinch of sea salt**
**pinch of cinnamon**
**½ cup apple juice**
**2 cups rolled oats**
**½ cup pastry flour**
**¼ cup coconut oil**
**2 teaspoons maple syrup**

Rinse and peel (or not) apples. Quarter and remove seeds. Place in a baking dish. Sprinkle with salt and cinnamon. Pour juice over the seasoned apples. Mix dry ingredients in a bowl and crumble over the apples. Gently press into the mixture. Bake at 350°F for 45 minutes until browned and apples are soft.

# DAY 10

## PLAY!

### *Recreation Will Re-create Your Body*

Moving your body is fun! It's a form of play. Think about a dog. Do you ever see how excited a dog gets when he knows he's going out for a walk? He starts to wag his tail, jump around, and pant with excitement—all from sensing that a fun routine is about to begin! Well, your body feels the same way. It's excited to move, and the time you set aside for movement is joyous! Unfortunately, many of us forget this as we grow up. Remember being a little kid and playing all day long? Those days were jam-packed with activities. During my childhood, I would go from one activity to the next: hide-and-seek, swimming, and competing in my dad's home-spun kid Olympics led to building forts, taking long walks, and pretending that I was going to set up house on an empty lot. After dinner, I

> *"It is a happy talent to know how to play."*
> — RALPH WALDO EMERSON

would get back outside with my best friend and finish the day by riding bicycles in circles into the night. By the end of the day, I felt exhausted, but it was as if every cell in my body was singing. The feeling of having used all of my physical energy, as well as my imagination, put me in a great mood and had me feeling relaxed and ready for sleep at the end of the day.

I took this notion of the joy of childhood play to heart on my twenty-fifth birthday. I wanted to have a special party, so I invited all of my friends to the park for a game of capture the flag. It was so great to watch my adult friends become children again. Being invested in the outcome, and strategizing just for the sake of fun, is so rare as we grow into adults. It was such a rush to get out my megaphone and shout out the rules, play a round of Simon says, and then let the games begin! The following day, and even two days later, I was getting calls from everyone telling me how sore they were and how wrecked their bodies felt. We are so out of practice with play that it is a workout!

If you cannot get a team sport together for this day, it's okay. Enjoy your time as if you were a child. If you were not very active, it's never too late. Now is the time to become childlike again. There are many activities you can do to put yourself into motion, get your heart rate up, and infuse your activity with the spirit of play. See the actions in this chapter for some ideas for bringing more play into today.

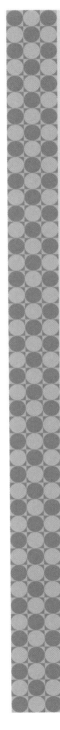

## ✣ ACTION CHECKLIST

**INTENTION:** *Recreation is re-creating my body.*

Exercise is creative and fuels my creativity. Creativity is the juice that fuels my exercise. I am a creative being.

**PLAYLIST:** *Dance to the Music*

This "play" list is just for playing around with different rhythms. Your heartbeat has a rhythm, your mind has a rhythm, and your breath has a rhythm. It seems your entire body is at play! You can use this or make your own fun playlist.

"Cut Chemist Suite," Ozomatli

"Girls & Boys," Prince

"Blister in the Sun," Violent Femmes

"Finally," Cece Peniston

"Do It ('Til You're Satisfied)," B.T. Express

"Knock On Wood," Amii Stewart

"Wild," Seal

"Peace Train," 10,000 Maniacs

"Under Pressure," Queen & David Bowie

"It's the End of the World as We
    Know It," REM

"Come A Long Way," Michelle Shocked

"Let My Love Open the Door," Pete
    Townshend

**YOGALOSOPHY ROUTINE VARIATION**

Blast party music. Or the daily playlist. Do the routine but in the spirit of play, create and have fun with it by making up your own poses and moves. Add one creative touch to each combo. Maybe it's a dance move, a twirl, or a somersault.

**CARDIO OPTION**

Do a fun activity. Remember the part of the body we want to focus on is the heart. The benefits of heart-rate training do not stop at the physical level. Yes, cardiovascular work is for our health, but the heart is also connected to our joy and love!

Here are some ideas for having fun through cardio activities:

- Rollerblade
- Jump rope
- Mini-trampoline
- Make up a dance routine and repeat it
- Hop or skip instead of walk

DAY 10

# POSES OF THE DAY

## Bridge, Wheel

### BRIDGE

Lie on your back with your knees bent at a ninety-degree angle, feet parallel on the floor and hip-distance apart. Take several breaths as you feel your body supported by the ground beneath you. Once you have settled in, press your feet evenly into the mat and lift your spine off of the floor, pressing your hips up as you root down through your feet. Scoop your tailbone under, and if you like, wriggle up onto the shoulders, interlacing the fingers and clasping the hands underneath you. Take five deep breaths. If you clasped the hands, unclasp them. Slowly lower down, one vertebra at a time.

Hug the knees into the chest to stretch the back.

**PHYSICAL BENEFITS:** Strengthens back, glutes, legs, and ankles. Opens chest, heart, and hip flexors. Stretches spine.

**HEALING BENEFITS:** Stimulates lungs, thyroid, and abdominal organs. Improves digestion.

**EMOTIONAL ASPECTS:** Energizes and lifts mood. Opens heart. Encourages vulnerability.

**MODIFICATIONS:** Place a yoga brick under your sacrum to support your lower back.

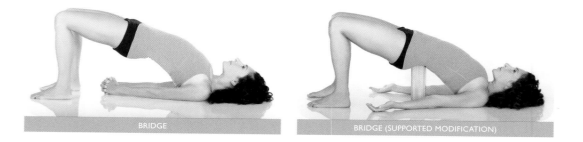

BRIDGE

BRIDGE (SUPPORTED MODIFICATION)

## WHEEL

Lie on the floor with your knees bent, and the soles of your feet hip-distance apart on the floor. Pull your heels close to your sit bones. Bend your elbows and place your hands on the floor next to your head, fingers spread and pointing toward your shoulder. Press your tail-bone up and lift your tush off of the floor. Keep thighs and feet parallel. Take three breaths. Press your feet and hands into the floor, inhale and, as you exhale, push away from the floor, straightening your arms. Rotate upper thighs inward and lengthen your tailbone toward the back of the knees. Spread the shoulder blades along the back and allow your head to hang. After a couple of breaths, slowly lower down by bending the elbows and tucking the chin. Hug your knees into your chest and rest.

PHYSICAL BENEFITS: Strengthens back and arms. Opens shoulders, chest, and spine.

HEALING BENEFITS: Helps asthma and some back pain. Stimulates thyroid, pituitary. Prevents osteoporosis.

EMOTIONAL ASPECTS: Lifts mood. Increases energy.

MODIFICATIONS: Bridge pose.

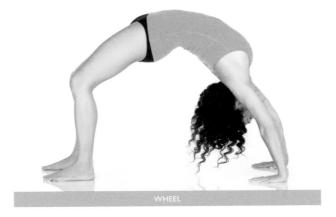

WHEEL

## EXTRA CREDIT: *Free your inner child!*

Do something fun today that breaks your routine and reminds you of being a child.

- See a play.

- Have a game night with friends.

- Screen a movie in your living room. Make popcorn and turn off all the lights.

- Build a fort in your living room.

- Pet an animal, or play catch with a child or fetch with a dog.

- Roll down a grassy hill!

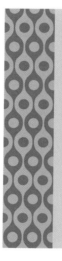

### ■ JOURNAL

Create a story today. Write something fictional and see what comes out. There is nothing more freeing than writing a fairy tale and creating fictional characters. They say that all of the roles in a play are simply different expressions of archetypes that reflect various aspects of ourselves. Enjoy the process and allow yourself to let go into it. Make yourself the main character and see where it leads.

### ■ GRATITUDE LIST

### ■ BREATHING EXERCISE

# Recipe: BANANA COCO COOKIES TO SHARE!

Make a healthy cake or bake cookies. Baking cookies makes me feel like a kid again. Here's a recipe I used recently.

**3 large, ripe well-mashed bananas (about 1½ cups)**
**1 teaspoon vanilla extract**
**¼ cup coconut oil, barely warm so it isn't solid (or alternately, olive oil)**
**2 cups rolled oats**
**⅔ cup almond meal**
**⅓ cup coconut, finely shredded and unsweetened**
**½ teaspoon cinnamon**
**½ teaspoon fine sea salt**
**1 teaspoon baking powder**
**6–7 ounces dairy-free, grain- or agave-sweetened chocolate chips or chopped dark chocolate**

Preheat oven to 350°F.

Place rack in the top third of the oven.

In a large bowl, combine the bananas, vanilla extract, and coconut oil. Set aside. In another bowl, whisk together the oats, almond meal, shredded coconut, cinnamon, salt, and baking powder. Add the dry ingredients to the wet ingredients and stir until combined. Fold in the chocolate chips/chunks. Drop dollops (about 2 teaspoons each) of the dough onto a baking sheet, an inch apart. Bake for 12–14 minutes.

Eat one cookie and share the rest.

# DAY 11

## CREATE HEALTHY HABITS
### *Self-care Builds Self-esteem*

**B**elieve me: No one likes routine less than I do. I wish that I could do my laundry just once and that would be it. Or take a final shower and be done with it for good. Sometimes routine is just plain boring! It's taken me a long time to understand that consistency and routine help me to be at my best. Maintaining a routine is essential to thriving, and it requires consistency. This is especially true of working out. I like to think of exercising as taking a shower from the inside out. Would you stop taking a shower or bath for an extended period of time? Of course not!

The point is that healthy habits make me feel great about myself. I'm not alone in my discovery about the success of routine. Any living thing thrives with consistency. A plant requires a certain amount of light and water on a regular basis. Children need routines for sleeping and eating. Even your pets need regimens for walks and mealtimes. In fact, there was a study of octogenarians that compared their lifestyles and how they lived so long. The one commonality was not what they ate or did physically, but that they had a consistent routine; they did the same thing at the same time every day. Try creating your own daily rituals and watch how quickly your body responds. I can't say that I can follow a routine for my entire life, but for this week, I can certainly create my own routine and see how the

*"A jug fills drop by drop."*
— BUDDHA

results feel. Even if I don't always follow it, I'll know what it feels like and know what works. You will find the same to be true.

One of my very favorite things about teaching is helping people to create healthy habits. The common thread among the celebrities I work with is a sense of commitment to their wellness routine. Kate Beckinsale, who is one of the most beautiful, healthy-looking, vibrant actresses I work with, insists on practicing yoga at least five times a week, and has extremely consistent eating habits. No matter how wealthy or famous or in love you are, no one else can exercise or eat well for you. You are in charge of caring for you. Everyone has a body that needs taking care of—and not just every now and then. Routine has helped me to stay tuned in to my body's needs. Think of your body as you would your car; it requires maintenance and fuel to keep in good working order. You would never just let a flashing light on your dashboard go on without addressing it, right? Yet when you have a pain in your body, you tend to ignore it, expecting it to disappear by itself. Often it takes an illness or an injury to bring people's attention back to the importance of healthy habits. After several injuries and years of practicing self-care, I now rest when I am tired, eat when I am hungry, and remind myself that getting the heart pumping blood to all my extremities, with my breath oxygenating my blood, is very important. The repetition becomes like a meditation on loving myself, and my body falls into place.

I'm not saying you have to get stuck in a monotonous rut, but it's important to remember that you become what you do daily. It's not the one piece of cake that you eat that causes weight gain, it's the two cookies you eat day after day. So go ahead and have a cookie! Then wake up the next morning—and the morning after—have a glass of warm water with lemon, meditate, take a walk, practice your yoga, have a healthy breakfast, and get back on the self-love train! If you do happen to go off, I have some detox tips to get you right back on track.

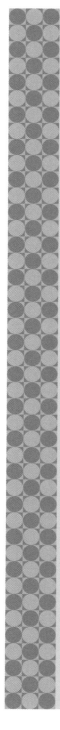

## ❧ ACTION CHECKLIST

### INTENTION: *"Detoxify."*

There is a lot of buzz these days around cleansing and detoxification. Let's get one thing straight: Even at your worst, you are not unclean or toxic. Your body is constantly restoring its natural balance all by itself. I am not a big advocate of long-term cleansing because the body wants balance, and if you do something long-term and extreme, you are likely to swing back the other way. This can become an endless cycle of punishment/reward. Then critical self-talk rears its head and says, "I am good when I am eating this way, and bad when I am not." Let's reboot by adding a detox element for today. But remember what is most important that you are detoxing: negative thinking.

### PLAYLIST: *Just Another Day*

This is one of my favorite mixes from my days as a spinning instructor. Working up a daily sweat has always been a part of my routine. I am sharing these optional playlists with you because these musical routines set the tone for the day.

"Woody and Dutch on the Slow Train to Peking," Ricki Lee Jones

"Magalenha," Sergio Mendes

"Spill the Wine," War

"Lonesome Day," Bruce Springsteen

"Grandma's Hands," Bill Withers

"Someday," The Strokes

"Boogie On Reggae Woman," Stevie Wonder

"Peace Train," Cat Stevens

"In My Place," Coldplay

"Sleepy Maggie," Ashley MacIsaac

"Semi-Charmed Life," Third Eye Blind

"Distractions," Zero 7

### YOGALOSOPHY ROUTINE VARIATION

Keep up with the Yogalosophy routine, or mix it up and try the detoxifying yoga routine included for today.

### CARDIO OPTION

Do ten Sun Salutations (see page 87) or twenty minutes of cardio, your choice. If you can get your hands on a mini-trampoline, jump on it for twenty minutes. It's amazing for your lymphatic system and will help you to detoxify.

DAY 11

# DETOXIFICATION GUIDELINES

**1** DETOXIFY THE MIND. First I recommend you lose toxic self-talk. Try taking on this new perspective: "Even if nothing changed, I have a perfect body." Believe it or not, it's true! Your body's natural state is health, and its job is to constantly eliminate what is no longer necessary. Embrace this stance to rid yourself of your negative perspective—even if only for a day.

This morning, start the day with a short meditation. This literally means five minutes of mindful breathing—simply inhale and exhale while paying attention to your breath. While doing this, set an intention. "I love my body exactly the way it is today" or "I am taking care of myself today." Imagine that on each inhale, you are replenishing yourself with life-force energy, and on each exhale you are expelling waste that is not needed.

**2** DETOXIFY YOUR EMOTIONS. To release stuck emotions, notice how you breathe. We established in an earlier chapter that the breath is the pathway from the mind to the body, and when you breathe, you are going to feel more. Breathing brings us into the present. Use this during your meditation or come back to this at the beginning of your practice or when you sit down to eat. During exercise, some emotions may come up, and they are all good, because that is your fuel. And that is what you have been suppressing with those desserts and sugary beverages. There is no judgment on negative and positive emotions; they are simply energy for you to use. The breath will eliminate what is no longer needed, which is alchemy for transforming your anger, grief, or even joy into pure energy.

**3** DETOXIFY YOUR BODY. Move your body to sweat it out. The mind/body union can happen during any physical activity, not just yoga. But try to integrate yoga into your walk, run, cycle, or elliptical routine by bringing intention and awareness of your body and breathing into all your exercise. Today is not the one time you are going to exercise. It is a routine you create because your body craves it. Follow my detoxifying routine, and you'll start seeing big changes!

# POSES OF THE DAY

## The Detoxifying Routine

Twists literally wring out the toxins from the body, while balance poses connect you with your core, and abdominal work targets and activates the midsection. Warm up with ten Sun Salutations, twenty minutes of cardio, or the Yogalosophy routine, and then embark on the following transformative detox routine. Hold each pose for five breaths.

PHYSICAL BENEFITS: Tones abdominals. Strengthens core and obliques.

HEALING BENEFITS: Aids digestion, wrings out toxins, encourages elimination.

EMOTIONAL ASPECTS: Reduces inertia. Increases energy, which inspires us to move toward our goals.

MODIFICATIONS: If you have any back injuries, avoid twists and replace them with the Yogalosophy routine. You will still detoxify by moving your body and breaking a sweat.

### THREE-LEGGED DOWNWARD FACING DOG

Come to your hands and feet, with your hands shoulder-distance apart and your feet about hip-width apart. Press your heels down as you lift your hips up. Shift your body weight forward toward your hands as you draw your right knee in toward your forehead. Engage your abs as you hold for five breaths.

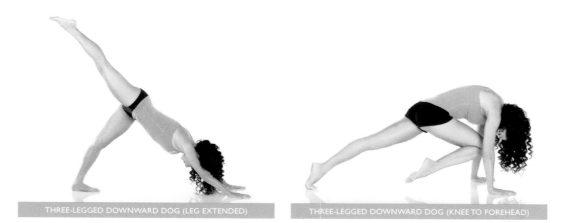

THREE-LEGGED DOWNWARD DOG (LEG EXTENDED)

THREE-LEGGED DOWNWARD DOG (KNEE TO FOREHEAD)

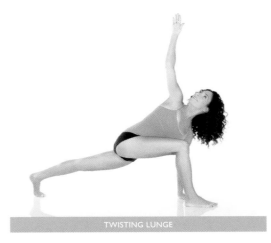

TWISTING LUNGE

### TWISTING LUNGE

Step your right foot forward between your hands and come up onto the ball of your left foot as you press your heel back. Try to straighten the left leg. Bring your left hand to the floor on the inside of your right foot. Twist your right arm up toward the ceiling and look up. Make sure your spine is extending from the tailbone through the crown of your head.

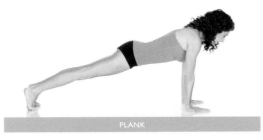

PLANK

### PLANK

Bring your right hand back down to the floor and step your right foot back to meet the left foot, staying up on your toes. Hold here in a high push-up position for three to five breaths. Move into Forearm Plank.

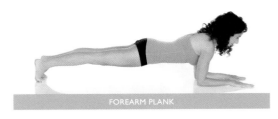

FOREARM PLANK

### FOREARM PLANK

Stay on your toes and slowly come down onto your forearms. This is where you will really need to stay connected to your core to keep your back straight. While here, lift your right foot off the floor just a couple of inches and hold using your abdominal muscles. Repeat on the left side. Press back up into Plank, then back to Downward Facing Dog.

## WARRIOR 3 TO EXTENDED LEG

From Downward Facing Dog, step your right foot through between your hands. Press gently off of the back leg and shift forward to balance on your right leg. Extend your arms out to the sides or back alongside your body. Balance here. Without putting your left foot on the floor, bring your hands to your hips, slowly hinge back up to standing and extend your left leg straight out in front of you.

## CHAIR AND CHAIR TWIST

With feet together, bend both knees and sit your hips back into an imaginary chair. Extend your arms up toward the ceiling, tuck your tailbone and use your core to lift your body away from the thighs. Bring your palms to a prayer position and hook the left elbow on the right knee. Press your palms together. Look up toward the ceiling. After holding for five breaths, unwind your body and go back to Downward Facing Dog. Repeat the sequence on the opposite side before transitioning to Boat Pose.

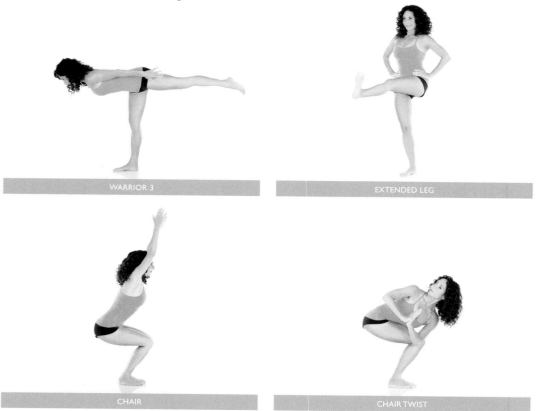

WARRIOR 3

EXTENDED LEG

CHAIR

CHAIR TWIST

BOAT

Balance on your sit bones and extend your legs upward and your arms out in front of you, parallel to the floor. If it is too challenging to keep your legs straight or if you have a lower back issue, you may bend the knees.

V-UPS

From boat, cross your arms over your chest and slowly lower your torso and legs down, using your abdominal strength. Hover with your feet and shoulders a couple of inches away from the floor. Then extend your arms and use your core to come back up to Boat.

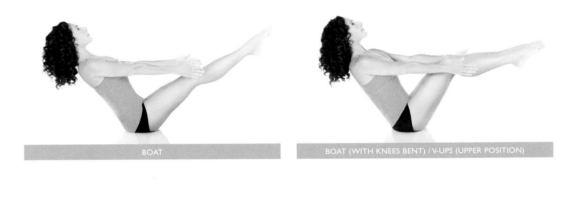

BOAT

BOAT (WITH KNEES BENT) / V-UPS (UPPER POSITION)

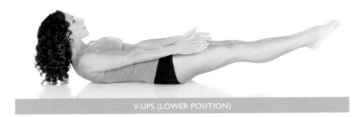

V-UPS (LOWER POSITION)

## SEATED TWIST

Bend your left knee on the floor in front of you. Cross your right leg over to bring your right foot to the outside of the left knee. Hook your left elbow on the outside of the right knee and press your right hand into the floor near the base of your spine. Inhale as you extend your spine up, then exhale as you twist back. Repeat on other side.

## RECLINING TWIST

Lying down on the floor, extend your arms out to the sides and bring your right foot on top of the left thigh. Slowly lower the right knee toward the left and look over your right shoulder. Relax into this twist. Repeat on other side.

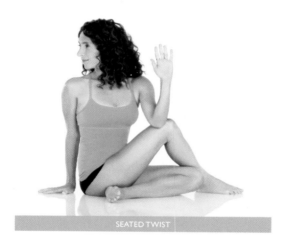

SEATED TWIST

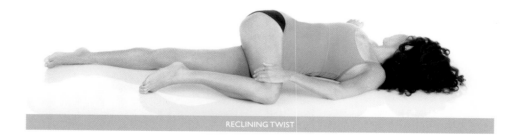

RECLINING TWIST

## EXTRA CREDIT: *Twenty-four-hour detox.*

Twice a year, I clean up my diet and do something a little challenging to reboot my system. This keeps me in my routine, but adds another level of fine-tuning and reminds me to be conscious that I am taking care of myself.

Even if you are not following the diet portion of the twenty-eight-day revolution, you can still eliminate one unhealthy food group from your diet and add one healthy replacement. It's always best, when removing something, to add something in its place. Examples: Eliminate coffee and replace it with green tea or eliminate sugar and replace with coconut water.

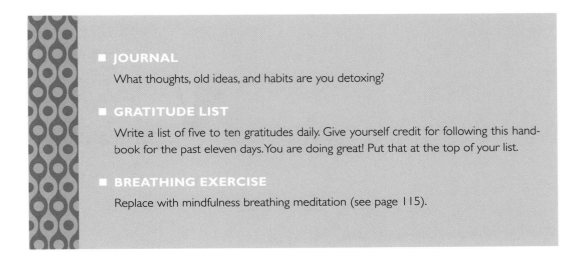

■ **JOURNAL**

What thoughts, old ideas, and habits are you detoxing?

■ **GRATITUDE LIST**

Write a list of five to ten gratitudes daily. Give yourself credit for following this handbook for the past eleven days. You are doing great! Put that at the top of your list.

■ **BREATHING EXERCISE**

Replace with mindfulness breathing meditation (see page 115).

# Recipe: ONE-DAY JUICE DETOX

This one-day cleanse is an experiment. The best way to look at it is as follows: You will have plenty of calories because you will be drinking juices. The purpose of a fast is to give your digestive system and your body a break. I do not personally recommend long fasts because the extreme reaction can swing you the other way.

This fast will include primarily vegetable juices, which you should drink five times a day (sixteen ounces per serving), as if it is your meal. Juice will load your body with nutrients while flushing your system.

The juices you drink should be fresh-pressed. You can either buy them at the store or blend yourself.

If you are not satisfied, feel free to drink more water. If you need an evening boost, drink coconut water.

## MORNING:

5 kale leaves

5 celery stalks

1 cucumber

1/2 cup parsley

1 piece ginger

1/2 lemon

## MIDMORNING:

1 cup spinach

4 kale leaves

1 lemon

1 cucumber

2 green apples

## LUNCHTIME:

5 kale leaves

1 cup spinach

2 stalks celery

1/2 apple

1/2 lemon

1/2 cup cilantro

1 piece ginger

## AFTERNOON:

juice of 3 lemons

water

spoonful of honey

cayenne pepper to taste

filtered water

## EVENING:

1 green apple

1 cup spinach

1/2 cup parsley

2 celery stalks

1 piece ginger

1/2 lemon

# DAY 12

## PRACTICE IMPERFECTLY

### You Already Have a Perfect Body

When I was first exposed to yoga as a child, I put a lot of pressure on myself to be perfect. I thought that having impeccable alignment, upper-body strength, unwavering balance, and gold-star breathing techniques would protect me from judgment and align me spiritually so that I would be untouchable, and I wouldn't have to feel afraid. More importantly, I would be loved and everyone would think I was amazing. I spent my teenage years seeking that level of greatness, especially in the external world. I consistently played the comparison game and would feel superior if I looked better than the person next to me and inferior if I envied their expertise.

> "If I wait until I become perfect before I love myself, I will waste my whole life. I am already perfect right here and right now. I am perfect exactly as I am."
>
> — LOUISE L. HAY

There was a point in my life, when I was about twenty, when my body looked the way I wanted it to look, the guy that I had an enormous crush on liked me too, I was excelling in my career as an actress, I had money, and I owned my own home. Everything on the outside seemed totally in place. You know the saying "Compare to no one but yourself"? That's what I did. But guess what? Some days I could not live up to what I did the day before, and I was having a hard time keeping up with myself. After I had achieved a certain level of perceived perfection, I felt the burden of maintaining it and could not feel safe. I felt afraid that what I had worked for would dissolve, and so I feared that I would lose it if I didn't keep juggling. I didn't realize then that life goes in cycles and things are not static, so perfection is a perception.

Ultimately, I learned to shift my naturally obsessive mind to finding perfection in the moment, not just the result. Being an instructor, this skill can still be awkward for me! However, what I have come to realize is that a teacher is simply a student who has taken the responsibility of being a guide. So what if I am imperfect! That's why feedback from the students is so vital. We are all finding our way together. It is my imperfections that allow my vulnerability and accessibility, both of which make me a better, more receptive, and relatable teacher.

This is part of the Y28 Revolution—you may be frustrated with imperfection. It's been twelve days now, and maybe your body isn't completely transformed, or your form is not in complete alignment. Don't worry. We all have times in our lives and our practices where we hesitate because we feel like we have to wait until we can execute with perfection. The good news is you don't have to wait! In fact, it's essential to your growth to feel challenged, uncomfortable, and like a beginner. Even if you're a longtime yoga practitioner, perhaps it's time to mix it up and become a beginner again. Whether you've gotten stuck in a rut doing the same classes again and again or are a newbie still learning the ropes, it's time to practice imperfectly!

Rather than focusing on the negative, observe yourself today; instead of trying to reach a specific goal, notice that your body has wisdom. If you follow its lead, you will be in the right place. You *are* in the right place.

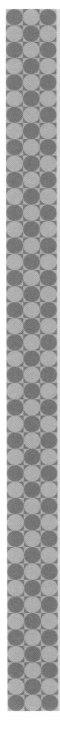

## ✣ ACTION CHECKLIST

### INTENTION: *Help others.*

When we stay overly focused on ourselves, it's very difficult to see change. Turning that attention outward, toward small favors we can do for others—from washing the dishes your roommate left in the sink to picking up your friend's daughter from school—will boost your self-esteem and allow you to place your focus on positive actions. "How can I be of service to others?" is a question you can ask yourself as you go through your day.

### PLAYLIST: *Heart-rate Training: Energy Up!*

Heart-rate training is a great way to purify your system by breaking a sweat. I created this playlist for one of my clients when they were training for an action movie, using today's cardio routine.

"Dance to the Music," Sly & the Family Stone

"Naughty Girl," Beyonce

"Headsprung," LL Cool J

"Vivrant Thing," A Tribe Called Quest

"Erotica," Madonna

"5-Piece Chicken Dinner," Beastie Boys

"Hey Ladies," Beastie Boys

"Shake Your Rump," Beastie Boys

"Subterranean Homesick Alien," Radiohead

### YOGALOSOPHY ROUTINE VARIATION

Add the abdominal routine (included in today's poses) between the two sets of Yogalosophy Routine poses.

### CARDIO OPTION

Opt for thirty minutes of your fave heart-rate-increasing exercise. I love to do this on an indoor bicycle, but you can do any favorite cardio activity. Alternate between pushing hard and a recovery pace. Pushing should be 90 percent of your maximum effort and recovery pace should be something you could maintain for a while, say 40 to 50 percent of your max.

- Start with five minutes recovery and a one-minute push.
- Then do two sets of three-minute recovery and one-minute push.
- Follow with two sets of two-minute recovery and one-minute push.
- Then alternate thirty seconds on, thirty seconds off, six times.
- Finish with a four-minute recovery and one-minute burst.

DAY 12

# POSES OF THE DAY

## Abdominal Routine

Abdominal exercises aid in heating up your body, increasing your metabolism, and improving your digestion. This will help you to digest information from all areas of your life. Do eight reps of each of the following nine exercises: Yogi Bicycles, Twisted Root Crunches, Lower Belly Lifts, Windshield Wipers, Heel Touches, Butterfly Pulses, Crunches, Reclining Splits with Pulses, Scissor Kicks

> PHYSICAL BENEFITS: Tones abdominals. This will help aid digestion and build heat in the body.
>
> HEALING BENEFITS: Aids digestion. Activates metabolism.
>
> EMOTIONAL ASPECTS: Connects with identity, sense of self, and desire.
>
> MODIFICATIONS: Use hands for support, behind both head and back.

### YOGI BICYCLES

Begin with knees hugged in to chest and hands behind head. Using abdominal strength, lift your upper body. Extend your right leg and cross your right elbow to the outside of the left knee. Exhale and draw the naval in toward the spine. Switch side to side for ten reps.

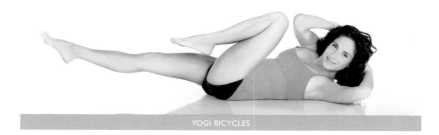

YOGI BICYCLES

## TWISTED ROOT CRUNCHES

Cross left leg over right and, if you are able, hook left foot behind right ankle. Wrap arms, right under left and, if possible, wind right hand around left wrist to bring your palms together. Curl upper and lower body simultaneously. Do ten reps. Switch sides and repeat.

## LOWER BELLY LIFTS

Extend legs up so that feet and hips are in alignment and your body is in an "L" shape, with arms by your sides. Use your lower abdominals and exhale as you press the feet straight up. The belly should draw in and down. Do ten reps.

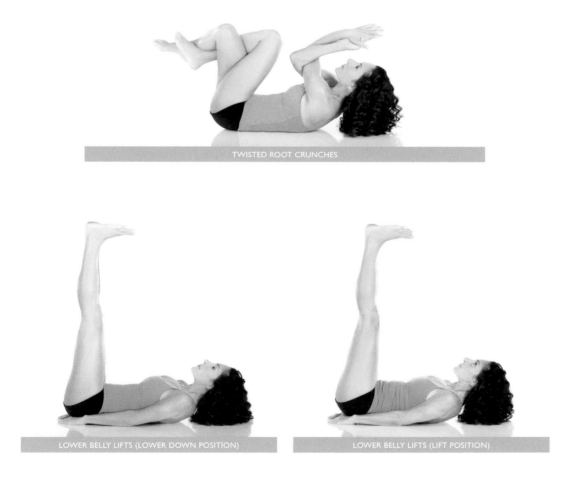

TWISTED ROOT CRUNCHES

LOWER BELLY LIFTS (LOWER DOWN POSITION)

LOWER BELLY LIFTS (LIFT POSITION)

## WINDSHIELD WIPERS

Recline and keep the heels above you, in line with your hips. Extend the arms out to the sides, shoulder level with the palms pressing down into the floor to brace you. Lower your straight legs halfway to the right, maintaining a connection to the abdominals. Use your ab strength as you bring the legs back and through to the other side. Repeat ten times. (Modification: bend knees but keep knees aligned with hips.)

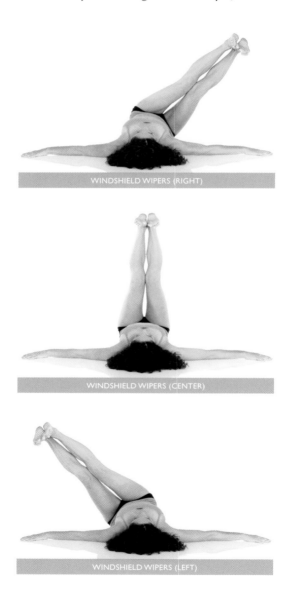

WINDSHIELD WIPERS (RIGHT)

WINDSHIELD WIPERS (CENTER)

WINDSHIELD WIPERS (LEFT)

## HEEL TOUCHES

Bring your feet apart on the floor, with knees pressing together. Reach down to your right heel and then to your left. Do side to side ten times.

## BUTTERFLY PULSES

Allow the knees to open to the sides and bring the heels together. Extend your arms and with palms together reach forward and pulse for ten reps.

## CRUNCHES

Plant the soles of your feet on the floor, hip-width apart. Place your hands behind your head and use your abdominal strength to lift. On the exhale, your upper body lifts as your naval draws down toward your spine. Do ten reps.

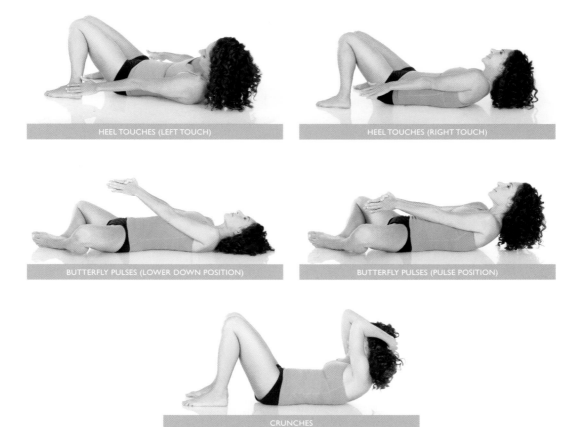

HEEL TOUCHES (LEFT TOUCH)

HEEL TOUCHES (RIGHT TOUCH)

BUTTERFLY PULSES (LOWER DOWN POSITION)

BUTTERFLY PULSES (PULSE POSITION)

CRUNCHES

## RECLINING SPLITS WITH PULSES

Extend your legs up and into a "V" split shape. Reach the arms between your legs and, with palms together, pulse through for ten reps.

## SCISSOR KICKS

Lift your hips and place your hands underneath you to ensure your lower back is on the floor (there should be no space between your lower back and the floor). Raise your torso up and scissor-kick your legs, one at a time. Do ten reps.

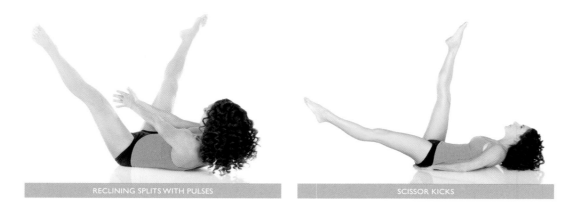

RECLINING SPLITS WITH PULSES          SCISSOR KICKS

## EXTRA CREDIT: *Try a new technique.*

Explore a new style of yoga and remember to PRACTICE IMPERFECTLY!

Here are some choices:

KUNDALINI: Since this yoga focuses on releasing the energy at the base of the spine, expect lots of breath work and moving energy along the spine. If you go to a class, don't be surprised if you see a turban or two, since this ancient yoga was developed by a Sikh guru.

HATHA: Most yoga postures are based on hatha, the "yoga of force." This means exerting effort. Many of the yoga postures we do in the Yogalosophy routine are based on hatha yoga poses, so it will feel familiar.

IYENGAR: This is the first yoga I tried and I love it for its alignment and form. B. K. S. Iyengar wrote the book *Light On Yoga*. It is a highly specific practice. Expect props, and be prepared to explore the right tip of your left kidney.

BIKRAM: This is the original "hot yoga," a series of twenty-six postures done two times in a row. The classroom is very hot, and students are discouraged from leaving the room or drinking for the first twenty minutes. However, nobody knows your body like you do, so you can override the teacher when it comes to evaluating what is best for you. These classes incorporate very little upper body work, which may appeal to people with wrist, neck, or shoulder issues. Be prepared to sweat—bring extra towels.

VINYASA: This practice focuses on flow yoga with Sun Salutations, stringing sequences of posture with the Salutations, and connecting movement with breath. It's the same as hatha but with a lot more movement, typically not holding postures for too long.

ANUSARA: Say hello to lots of heart-opening and backbends. This is yoga for the heart, and one I have never tried due to a couple of herniations in my spine, so I would be practicing imperfectly with you!

YIN YOGA: Much more stretchy and slow, this passive yoga can be great for type A personalities to unwind and be softer, unraveling and dissolving all the thinking that you do.

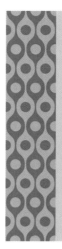

■ **JOURNAL**

What is a flaw of yours that became a strength?

■ **GRATITUDE LIST**

List three things about yourself that are already perfect. List three things that are flaws. Yes! Be grateful for your flaws. In your practice (and we know what practice makes), remind yourself that this is already exactly as it should be.

■ **BREATHING EXERCISE**

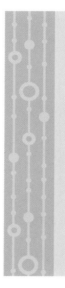

## *Recipe:* FRESH INGBER TEA
### (INGBER IS GINGER IN YIDDISH AND GERMAN!)

This helps digestion, wards off colds, and is an anti-inflammatory. In short, it's really, really good for you. Enjoy.

**4 cups filtered water**
**2-inch piece fresh gingerroot**
**Optional: honey, lemon**

Peel the gingerroot and thinly slice. Bring water to a boil in a saucepan, then add ginger. Simmer for 15–20 minutes. Strain. Add honey and lemon to taste.

# DAY 13

## CULTIVATE A RELATIONSHIP WITH YOUR BODY

### *Yoga Means Union*

Your body is your primary relationship. Lovers come and go, friends can drift apart, children grow up and leave, parents pass away, and coworkers and workplaces change. The only guaranteed constant for this lifetime is your amazing vehicle of a body. That's why developing a healthy relationship with it is even more important than the relationship you have with your friends, partner, children, and parents. If you are putting everyone and everything else before your body, you are missing out on the greatest and most intimate and important relationship of your life!

Over the years, I have had many different types of relationships with my body. I have often treated myself like an abusive lover, conditional and unforgiving, demanding that I whip myself into shape with punishment. I have been a patient mother, sitting with injuries and nursing them as they heal. I have even been my own best friend, reminding myself by listing the things that I love about my body. With all the ups and downs, I have often thought I am my own worst boyfriend, and I have tried but I just can't seem to break up with me. So I may as well commit.

> *"When you truly give up trying to be whole through others, you end up receiving what you always wanted from others."*
>
> — SHAKTI GAWAIN

133

Marriage, I hear, is not easy and requires work. Staying in a healthy relationship with yourself is similar. To feed my commitment, each day I take a loving action toward myself by keeping my fitness vows. A loving commitment to my body, whether I feel like it or not, gives me the self-respect I deserve. I know that it's enough to just show up for myself and express my gratitude by using and moving my limbs. I communicate with my body, asking what is okay and modifying when necessary. Feeling, sensing, playing, and enjoying the re-creation of my body. I get to utilize my own attention to detail, and lovingly work on my nature without judgment or attachment to the result. Through cleansing, purifying, and creating a routine that keeps me balanced through turbulent times, I experience alchemical and inner transformation just by hanging in there!

My body's breakdowns and breakthroughs give me more experience, which leads to self-mastery and authority over my own body. I then get to widen my scope by sharing with my community all that I have learned as part of my spiritual practice. That is what it is to be married to your body. That is the twenty-eight-day revolution process you have committed to with this program.

Today be your own ideal mate. Treat yourself the way you want to be treated. Notice the way you speak to yourself, and how that relationship is when you are practicing yoga. Yoga is an effective way to reconnect and get intimate with all parts of yourself.

The word yoga means "union." It describes the union of the masculine and feminine parts of yourself, of mind/body and spirit, of the universal spirit and self. As above, so below. As you strive to unite your opposites, remember that the yogic path is really a path of "both/and" rather than "either/or."

I am a blend of my original male and female prototypes. I have my father's drive, but also his temper. I have my mother's kindness and humor, but also her defensiveness. I try to integrate all facets of myself from within. I find that when I can accept both the dark and the light, the joy and the grief, as two sides of the same coin—not able to see one another, yet not able to survive alone—I can start to understand my own base nature and can at last accept all of who I am. The more I do that, the more access I have to balance. That is true commitment. The balance of opposites is the key.

## ✻ ACTION CHECKLIST

### INTENTION: *Embrace your opposites.*

The mission of this day is inspired by the sometimes paradoxical relationship between our different sides. The push/pull of opposites can be confusing without the acceptance that there is more than one aspect to yourself. You can want more than one thing at the same time. You can be both happy and longing. You can be selfish and a giver. Settling into your own skin and owning the seductress as well as the little girl, or the warrior and the damsel-in-distress, means that you are free to be all of who you are, without apology. Honor all of it. Celebrate it. Commit fully to all aspects of you.

### PLAYLIST: *It Takes Two*

Enjoy this selection of duets!

"Two of Us," Aimee Mann & Michael Penn

"Cecilia," Simon and Garfunkle

"I've Got You, Babe," Sonny & Cher

"Give It to Me," Timbaland (featuring Nelly Furtado & Justin Timberlake)

"Don't Give Up," Peter Gabriel and Kate Bush

"Don't Let the Sun Go Down on Me," Elton John & George Michael

"Ain't No Mountain High Enough," Marvin Gaye & Tammi Terrel

"Sara," Daryl Hall & John Oates

### YOGALOSOPHY ROUTINE VARIATION

Imagine that exercise is a courtship. A dance of give and take. Do not force yourself. Allow, allow, allow. Add the following balance options to the Yogalosophy routine:

For the Chair pose, balance on tiptoe for a couple of breaths.

When you Plié Squat, do the same.

After the Lunges, add Warrior 3 and Half Moon Pose (today's pose). Then move back into the lunge and transition back into the routine.

### CARDIO OPTION

Ask yourself today what you would like to do. Listen. And do that.

DAY 13

# POSES OF THE DAY

## Warrior 3, Half Moon

Balance is not stillness, but it is harnessing dynamic energy, which is in constant flux. The two forces extending in opposite directions are very active and require your focus and presence. For instance, if you are thinking while in a balance pose, you will likely topple over. Remember: Energy flows where the mind goes, so if you are making your grocery list in your mind, your energy is at the market. These balances are tricky, so use the pose modifications if you need to at first. Don't worry. Before you know it, you'll be balancing on your own.

Below are the top three tips to help with balance:

**1** FIND A GAZING POINT. They say when the gaze is still, the mind is still. Find a point of focus that does not move, then fix your gaze.

**2** BREATHE. When you focus on your breath and the natural rhythm of your body, the mind begins to relax. The mind needs a focus, so the breath can be a centering rhythm.

**3** EXTEND. Balance comes from extension. So think of a line of energy running through your body extending in both directions. If palms are touching, press them together; pushing against also implies two opposite forces.

### WARRIOR 3

Begin in Crescent pose (see Yogalosophy Routine, page 9). Interlace the fingers behind the back and pull the shoulders down and away from the ears. Find a gazing point and fix your gaze. As you focus on your breath, shift your weight onto your front leg and lean forward until your leg and torso are on the same line, like the letter T. Make sure your standing leg is straight and find extension out through the crown of the head and the back extended heel. Breathe, and if you feel comfortable, reach the arms forward by your ears.

PHYSICAL BENEFITS: Tones abs, strengthens legs.

HEALING BENEFITS: Improves balance and posture. Focuses mind.

EMOTIONAL ASPECTS: Lifts mood. Increases energy.

MODIFICATIONS: Place a chair in front of you and practice using it as needed.

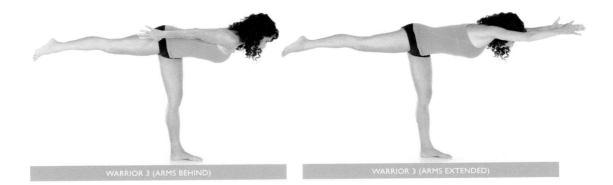

WARRIOR 3 (ARMS BEHIND)

WARRIOR 3 (ARMS EXTENDED)

## HALF MOON POSE

A refresher on this pose: From Crescent pose, lower your right fingertips to the floor, six inches in front of your right pinky toe. Stack the hips on top of each other as you extend your left arm up to the sky. Open the chest to the ceiling as much as you can, so that the head, hips, shoulders, and heels are in alignment. After several breaths, bring your left hand to the floor and step back into a lunge. Resume the Yogalosophy routine.

PHYSICAL BENEFITS: Balance. Strengthens abs, thighs, and glutes. Tones lower back muscles.

HEALING BENEFITS: Improves digestion.

EMOTIONAL ASPECTS: Focuses the mind and brings you into the present moment. Relieves anxiety and fatigue.

MODIFICATIONS: Use a wall, chair, or block for support as needed.

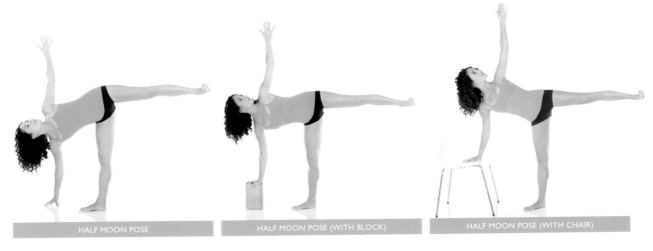

HALF MOON POSE

HALF MOON POSE (WITH BLOCK)

HALF MOON POSE (WITH CHAIR)

## EXTRA CREDIT: *Make an altar.*

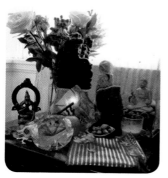

Create a sacred space that symbolizes various aspects of yourself. I like to include objects that honor all facets of my spirit: the lover, the mother, the child, and God. Even my weaknesses get a seat at the altar. When you invite all of yourself in, you bring the darker sides into the light of consciousness, illuminating your whole self.

An altar does not have to be religious. You can honor any masters you admire—from poets and prophets to inspirational leaders—by including quotes or writing that reflect their wisdom. You can also include objects from nature that remind you of sacred moments, like seashells or stones, a found feather or crystal, but each item should be empowering for you. You can add carved figures or artifacts, even photos of special moments—anything that represents your sacred self. You can also offer fruit, flowers, and chocolate at your altar!

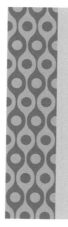

■ **JOURNAL**

Write a love letter to yourself.

■ **GRATITUDE LIST**

Make a "Love Yourself" list. Write down at least five things you love about your body—both the perfect and the imperfect.

■ **BREATHING EXERCISE**

*Recipe:* **NO COOKING TODAY!**

Take yourself out. Stay on the eating plan when you order!

# DAY 14

## CELEBRATE YOUR BEAUTY

### Fall in Love with Yourself

You are already such a beautiful being, and you know this because as you look around, you can see that there is beauty in everything around you. This beauty is a reflection of what you hold inside. Everything is a reflection of ourselves. If you see beauty, it is because you are beautiful. But what if you don't see beauty? What if when you look around, you do not see what is grace, but instead you see the negative, the less-than-perfect?

It's time to retrain your eyes and get some rose-colored glasses. When you see a roly-poly puppy whose stomach drags on the ground, you certainly are not thinking how ugly and fat that little dog is, but how adorable that being is. Begin to notice the beauty and grace all around you all the time. There is a dance of life that is perfectly timed and choreographed. Notice what graces your presence, and pay attention to lucky events that unfold before you. The universe is sending you little miracles and gifts all the time.

> "Loving yourself is the key to loving others. Love begins with you."
>
> — DON MIGUEL RUIZ

Bringing more beauty into your environment will help to reinforce your awareness of beauty and the feeling of grace and balance. You don't have to spend a lot of money to do this. Lighting some candles and putting on some classical music will immediately shift the energy in your environment. I love Bach and when I play that music, I feel uplifted. Even the flicker of the candle appears to move to the music when I pay attention to the dance of synchronicities all around me.

Buy yourself some flowers and pay attention to your own physical presentation today. Walk with your spine straight and dress in clothes that make you feel good, something that hugs your curves and feels loose and flowy—a fabric that is soft to the touch.

Remember that beauty is about perspective. There is no one quite like you. You are a unique individual, and you are the perfect fit for you. Plus, you have an inner beauty all of your own that emanates and radiates from within. Notice what is already beautiful about your body today. Try paying attention to what is special and lovable about you. Stretching and extending beyond your perception is beauty in and of itself.

I just got an opportunity to look at my beauty in a new way. I was asked to model in some yoga stretches for German *Vogue*. I put it on my to-do list, never giving it a second thought until the day approached and I got my call sheet. The list of photographers, hair and makeup artists, assistants, and the word *Vogue* plastered all over this document, jarred me into reality and it suddenly occurred to me that I was going to be a model in a beauty magazine. Impossible! Beneath all of my sweetness, confidence, and power, there is an insecure girl who feels she misses the mark on the beauty standard. When I have been complimented on my looks, I have shunned it, declaring that part of the reason I am special is BECAUSE I don't look like a model. I have blown it off as if it hasn't mattered in the least, but when this photo shoot came up, I felt like I was realizing a little girl dream that I never even allowed myself to have. This caused me to see that my own beauty standard is slowly changing. Certainly when I was a girl, if I had declared that I wanted to model, there would be a lot of good reasons for my mother to steer me in a different direction. I am glad today that I am not asking for anyone's permission. I see now that slowly, my view of my own beauty has shifted. The most surprising element about the photo shoot was they weren't trying to make me look any different than I am. They were not trying to change me, but were looking to capture my inner beauty.

You deserve to be acknowledged for the inner beauty you possess. If you are like I am and your default tends toward self-criticism, do what I do and err on the side of effusive self-love. I find this balances my self-defeating tendencies and should do the same for you! Embody that with a balance pose. Finding balance can literally help to extend your reach beyond your immediate physical body, without disrupting the space around you. Balance is about extension. It's even about finding another dimension of tension, which is dynamic and alive. This fiery aliveness of your own is a true celebration!

## ✕ ACTION CHECKLIST

### INTENTION: *Love yourself.*

Loving yourself won't take anything away from anyone else. In fact, it is contagious. Face it, there's no one who gets your jokes like you do, you don't have to wonder what you are thinking, or wait for yourself to call. This commitment is 100 percent and there's nothing you have to hide from you. Imagine the love you are looking for and give it to yourself.

### PLAYLIST: *The Love Mix*

I have made many a love mix. Use mine, or make your own "Love Yourself" playlist.

"My Heart, My Life," Nusrat Fateh Ali Khan

"Love Is Alive," Gary Wright

"Feelin' Love," Paula Cole

"Damn I Wish I Was Your Lover," Sophie
   B. Hawkins

"Where Is the Love," Black Eyed Peas

"Love to Be Loved," Peter Gabriel

"Bold as Love," Jimi Hendrix

"Lover Lay Down," Dave Matthews Band

"Your Love Is King," Sade

"Give Me Love," George Harrison

"Love and Affection," Joan Armatrading

"I Can't Make You Love Me," George
   Michael

"Romeo and Juliet," Dire Straits

### YOGALOSOPHY ROUTINE VARIATION

Be fluid and graceful with the Y28 movements. Treat the session like it is a ballet class and even play classical music. Make sure to lengthen your limbs by pointing your toes. If you feel inclined to twirl, please do so.

### CARDIO OPTION

Take a dance class, or do a pretend thirty-minute ballet class. Favor long, sweeping movements over sweat today. Stay balanced and self-possessed. Never let them see you sweat.

DAY 14

# POSE OF THE DAY

## DANCER'S POSE

Begin in Mountain pose. Standing straight up, find a gazing point of stillness. Bend your right elbow and hinge your arm out to the right. Bend your right leg behind you by curling your heel up toward your tush. With your right hand, hold your right arch from the inside. Extend your left arm up by your left ear, and inhale. On the inhale, fix your gaze and keep the standing leg very straight and reach forward with your left extended arm. Press the top of the back right foot into the hand and lean forward. Keep drawing the right knee back behind you. You will feel a great stretch on the right shoulder and lower back, as well as your legs. Come out of this as gracefully as you got into it and switch sides. Hold each side for five breaths or thirty seconds.

PHYSICAL BENEFITS: Stretches shoulders, hips, groin, inner thigh, and abdomen. Strengthens legs and ankles.

HEALING BENEFITS: Improves balance and focus. Good for kidneys, spine, and lungs.

EMOTIONAL ASPECTS: Creates emotional balance, energizes, and elevates mood.

MODIFICATIONS: Use a wall to brace yourself. Don't lean forward as deeply.

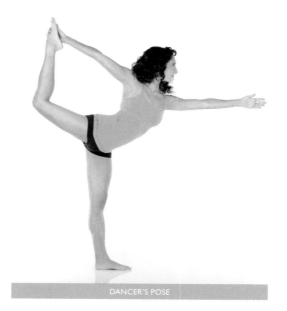

DANCER'S POSE

## EXTRA CREDIT: *Romance yourself.*

Take yourself on a date.

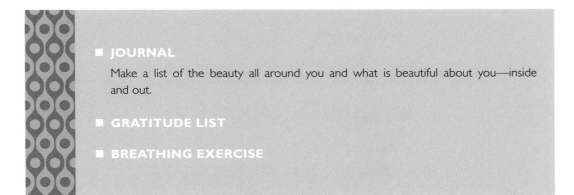

- **JOURNAL**

  Make a list of the beauty all around you and what is beautiful about you—inside and out.

- **GRATITUDE LIST**

- **BREATHING EXERCISE**

## *Recipe:* STRAWBERRY SPRITZER

Celebrate your beauty with a non-alcoholic glass of bubbly.

1 champagne glass
2 strawberries
1 cup sparkling water

Trim and halve the strawberries. Fill champagne flute with sparkling water, drop in strawberries, and enjoy!

# DAY 15

## BREAK ON THROUGH

### *The Moment You Want to Give Up Is the Moment Your Body Is Changing*

**R**ight about now you may be thinking you've done enough, why not just stop here? Or take a break? Usually, about halfway through a process like this, that voice will come up. So if that's what you are saying to yourself right now, if that voice is whispering (or shouting) in the back of your mind, it means you are on the right track! A revolution can't happen without a revolt!

> *"Courage faces fear and thereby masters it."*
>
> — MARTIN LUTHER KING, JR.

The moment you feel that you want to give up is the exact point on the path where the breakthrough muscle gets stronger. It is almost as if that mechanism is built into you like internal willpower weights, or resistance bands of intention. Every moment that you experience the desire to quit and you do not, you exercise and strengthen that voice within you that says "yes." You invigorate your self-esteem and the fighter in you. It's true. Of course, it's nice to feel safe and comfortable, but staying comfortable is not the place of change. That intense period of discomfort is the moment your body is changing. So move toward the intensity.

When you push through, you literally give your body a new cellular memory. It is now a proven fact that the observer changes the experiment, so when you think you can't do it, watch your thoughts and change the experiment. That's just your mind, so choose a new thought. This is where all of the tools you have been sharpening so far come into play.

When I am struggling with something that feels impossible, I call upon the genetic history that is literally in my body, blood, and bones. I go back to connecting with my grandfather: Sasha Lipshutz (or in America, Sam Lipszyc). When I feel like I want to quit, I remember his story.

At age seventeen, my grandfather escaped from Poland, leaving behind his mother, sister, and four brothers, who were killed in the Holocaust. He and his half-brother made a run for it into a potato field, and although he was stabbed in the back attempting to run, he escaped a concentration camp. He traveled to Russia, where he met my grandmother in a coal mine while he was working on a rescue team. They fell in love, and he built a cabin in Siberia with his own hands, where my uncle was born. Somehow he and my grandma survived the horrors of war and ended up in a displaced persons camp in Germany, where they had my mother. The family immigrated to the United States via relatives in Chicago and ended up in Los Angeles, California, where Sam Lipszyc worked hard to rebuild his life, starting his own business building parts for planes and rocket ships.

All of that just so I could be born in L.A. and have such problems as worrying about not being invited to a party, my boyfriend not returning my call, or gaining seven pounds. I am joking, of course. I never worry about my boyfriend calling me back. We are made of stronger stuff than we realize. You have a story too. When you really go back and imagine all of the struggles that your ancestors went through so that you can be right here, working on your body, mind, and spirit, it is truly awesome. And that very strength is within your DNA.

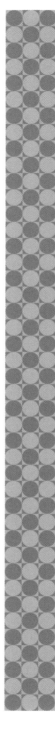

## ✕ ACTION CHECKLIST

### INTENTION: *Bring it on!*

"If this action gets me closer to my goal, then BRING IT ON!"

### PLAYLIST: *America Playlist*

This playlist is in honor of my grandfather. I always tell his story in my class when I play "America" by Simon & Garfunkel.

"America," Neil Diamond

"American Woman," Lenny Kravitz

"American Baby," Dave Matthews Band

"American Girl," Tom Petty & The Heartbreakers

"Young Americans," David Bowie

"White America," Eminem

"America," Simon & Garfunkel

"America, Fuck Yeah," Team America

"American Pie," Don McLean

"American Idiot," Green Day

"Ventura Highway," America

### YOGALOSOPHY ROUTINE VARIATION

This is a day to build to a breaking point. Do the "fully loaded" fifty-five minute routine today (see the Yogalosophy Extras in the back of the book). It's a long one, but once you get over this hurdle, you are halfway home. Here's what it includes:

Fully Loaded 55-Minute Routine

- Sun Salutations (page 231)
- Strength Series (page 233)
- Balance Challenge (page 234)
- Yogalosophy Poses/Toners (page 9)
- Stretch (page 236)

### CARDIO OPTION

Do a high-intensity aerobic activity today for at least thirty minutes. Try a spinning class (see extra credit) or do a cross-fit workout. Yes, that's two hardcore workouts today. There are no other days like today in this Y28 day Revolution. Take it!

DAY 15

# POSES OF THE DAY

YOGALOSOPHY EXTRAS (SEE PAGE 230)

PHYSICAL BENEFITS: Endurance work. Incorporates strength, balance, and stretching.

HEALING BENEFITS: Changes your DNA by bringing you beyond your threshold.

EMOTIONAL ASPECTS: Transcending what you have already done will bring self-confidence and emotional strength.

MODIFICATIONS: If you are ill today, sit it out. Otherwise, modify accordingly. Just do what you can.

## EXTRA CREDIT: *Ride it out.*

Take a spinning class or go for a bike ride. Pedal hard!

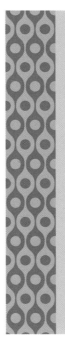

■ **JOURNAL**

Breakthrough or breakdown—what is the voice that carries you through? Option to journal about the story of your ancestors and how you got right here.

■ **GRATITUDE LIST**

List five things you have inherited from your ancestors that have made you strong.

■ **BREATHING EXERCISE**

■ **DIET MODIFICATION:** *Week 3*

- Keep Going!
- Add a twenty-minute walk in the evening after dinner.
- Chew your food well.
- Think gratitude each time before you eat.

## *Recipe:* BUBBIE'S MASHED POTATO KUGLE

My grandmother is eighty-eight years old and still alive. She suggests you hand shred the potatoes and onions. She showed me the shredder and it is the same one I remember her using forty years ago. My mother suggested a food processor, but Bubbie Sonia claims it will not be the same. Bubbie knows best.

**5 medium potatoes**
**5 eggs**
**1 medium onion**
**pinch of salt**
**canola (or coconut) oil**

Hand shred potatoes and drain the liquid. In a separate bowl, hand shred the onions and drain the liquid. Add eggs and onions to potato mixture. Add salt to taste. In a large skillet, add enough oil to cover pan and heat on a high flame. With a large serving spoon, scoop a dollop of the mixture and fry in pan. Makes 10 pancakes. Share with family.

# DAY 16

## TRANSFORM

### *Lean Into the Darkness*

Transformation does not come without a hero's journey into the dark. Alchemy does not happen without getting burned, and you do not truly change until you have faced your dark night of the soul. The Adyashanti quote below, which I added to my own vision board, says that you need to own the dark as a part of the self. When darkness is projected as something "out there," it appears to victimize you through circumstance. When you own it, it can actually be the seat of great empowerment.

I, like most people, am a feel-good junkie. Why else would I be attracted to a job where I wear comfortable clothes and no makeup, and lead people to the ultimate moment:

*"Make no mistake about it—enlightenment is a destructive process. It has nothing to do with becoming better or being happier.*

*Enlightenment is the crumbling away of untruth. It's seeing through the façade of pretense. It's the complete eradication of everything we imagined to be true."*

— ADYASHANTI

Savasana, where they get to float off into bliss for five to ten minutes? This is the "yoga" that we all imagine, right? Hugs and sitting peacefully in a cross-legged position with no earthly desires. But make no mistake, in order for us to transcend, the part of ourselves that is addicted to being comfortable must die and be replaced with the part of ourselves that demands growth. There is no growth without change, and there is no change without discomfort.

How can we reframe these old ideas we have about the sensations that we label "torture"? Perhaps to spin the old "I'm dying!" into "I know this is my body transforming" or "if this difficulty takes me closer to my goal, then bring it on!"

Much like the reference to enlightenment in the Adyashanti quote, the physical transformation process is also a destructive process. You are literally breaking down the muscles, which causes your body to rebuild and get stronger. If you own this breakdown as part of the process rather than making yourself a victim to it, you will find an incredible power that is breaking through from within. That is where all of the alchemy is. You will see that when you get more involved and confront the feeling, your task will actually become easier, and you will feel stronger. Sometimes it is this place of intimacy that you must treat like surgery. Go in, laser-like and focused, finding a way to connect with your power to transform. Hang in there. When the endorphins kick in, it's like a natural anesthesia. The shape of your body will change, and you will know that you are actively involved in this alchemy as you hit that uncomfortable edge and feel that burn. Do not shy away from that feeling, move toward that pain threshold, because this is the feeling of transformation.

It was Jennifer Aniston who told me this parable about how a pearl is created. This is how it happens. A grain of sand gets stuck inside the shell of an oyster. The oyster is so uncomfortable with the grain of sand that it tries to push it out, which only creates more of an irritant. As the oyster keeps trying and trying to force it out, the grain of sand has finally become a shining pearl. Then, when someone tries to pry the pearl out of the oyster, the oyster holds on for dear life to this precious jewel it has created through its struggle. This also reminds me of a funny saying: A diamond is just a piece of coal that hung in there. I love these stories because I can relate to irritations and pressures, which can be catalysts for creating something beautiful.

Your struggle is beautiful! Much like the phoenix rising from the ashes of destruction, you will hit a point of transformation and alchemy when you will soar above your former self and your current situation to be reborn. Using another jewel analogy, when I am working out with intensity, I think of melting gold down so that it can be reshaped and made into another beautiful piece. I just allow myself to move through the pain willingly. And the next day, I often wake up peaceful and happy; I feel different because I know that I have changed for the better, simply by enduring the feeling of change as it occurs. That's the gift.

Going through something very challenging and difficult can become the source of your awesome power. The workout is a great place to experiment with this edge. I have learned from and used it as a template for how to survive a break up, my father's passing, and loss of a job that I loved. The physical reality is a wonderful teacher for even deeper moments when we must endure emotional and psychic pain with grace and equanimity.

There are many instances, even during a difficult yoga practice, when you want to shy away and give up. Those are the moments of discomfort that are so incredibly intimate when you actually begin to find yourself. When you are in the transformative process, the darkness that you come up against is the closest you come to your most powerful self. You must face that darkness in order to access all of who you are. Yes, it is scary to do, but it beats the alternative of running away. In facing your own darkness, you experience true faith in the transformative process. That level of trust and intimacy is the empowering moment.

Empowerment is the result of coming through the other side of loss. You are losing something right now: that comfortable feeling, old habits, procrastination, and stagnation. You have had to take the time and put in the effort daily, and you have chosen to restrict yourself so that you can be right here today. YES! YES to the struggle. YES to the discomfort! YES to all of it. You are in the most pivotal part of the journey. In your hero's journey, you are at the peak of your personal arc, and you are all in.

Nice to meet you.

## ✕ ACTION CHECKLIST

**INTENTION:** *Transcend.*

Without pain, there is no change. When you truly accept where you are, you will begin to transcend the feeling of pain. One of the most beneficial aspects of yoga is learning how to find that threshold and move toward it, rather than shy away from it. In order to truly transcend, the very darkness we resist must be embraced. The part of ourselves that wants to be comfortable must die and be replaced with the part of ourselves that demands growth. There is no growth without change, and there is no change without discomfort.

**PLAYLIST:** *The Dark Mix*

This is a high-intensity mix. You don't have to like it; you just have to get through it, if you choose.

"Cups," Underworld

"Battleflag," Lo Fidelity Allstars

"L.A. Woman," The Doors

"Freedom," George Michael

"Angry Anymore," Ani DiFranco

"Silence," Delerium

"Can't Find My Way Home," Blind Faith

"Walk this Land," E-Z Rollers

**YOGALOSOPHY ROUTINE VARIATION**

What doesn't kill you makes you stronger, more focused, and laser-sharp. Push your edge. Push yourself to a rebirth. Add Sun Salutations, five push-ups, and five minutes of cardio bursts between each exercise in your Yogalosophy routine.

**CARDIO OPTION**

The cardio bursts in the routine should do it for you. If not, retread the idea of that spinning class.

DAY 16

# POSE OF THE DAY

### EAGLE POSE

Begin with your feet together. Inhale, sweep your arms up overhead, and on the exhale, swing them down to hook your right elbow under your left elbow. Twist your arms like a cinnamon twist (make it gluten-free!), and place your palms together if you can. Cross your right leg over your left leg and, if possible, wrap your right foot behind your left ankle. Bend your knees and sink your hips back, as if you are sitting back into a chair. Raise your wrapped arms up, so that your elbows are in front of your face. Your tendency may be to swivel your hips to the right, so shift them back to neutral. Hold for five breaths.

PHYSICAL BENEFITS: Strengthens legs and shoulders, improves balance, focus, and concentration.

HEALING BENEFITS: Opens the joints. Increases blood flow to reproductive organs and kidneys.

EMOTIONAL ASPECTS: Balances emotions. Reduces tension.

MODIFICATIONS: If you cannot wrap the foot around the calf, just cross the leg over. Or do Tree Pose (see page 50).

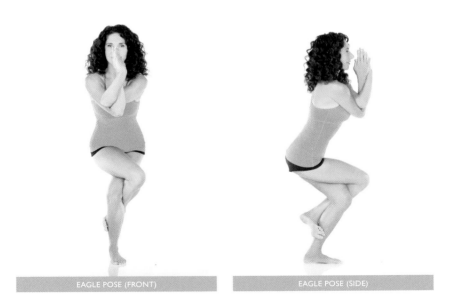

EAGLE POSE (FRONT)                    EAGLE POSE (SIDE)

## EXTRA CREDIT: *Push your boundaries.*

The five advanced power moves below are meant to push the envelope a little. Avoid forcing, but try to allow your body to go a little farther than you thought possible and notice what happens to your mind as your metamorphosis begins and you transform. The key to going deeper is not to push past the pain or to force your body, but to tolerate the feeling by staying with it rather than backing off. Once you have surrendered to the feeling, the body will settle in and transcend it without effort.

### KING PIGEON

Sitting on the floor, bend your right knee in front of you and bring your left leg behind you in a straight position. The heel of your right foot is in toward your left hip. Make sure to rotate the left hip down, so that the front of your left thigh is on the floor.

For the next stage of this posture, moving into King Pigeon, it is important that your spine and shoulders are warmed up. Bend your left leg, so that the toes are pointing up toward the ceiling. Take hold of the foot with your left hand, arch your back, and slide the toes of your left foot into the crease of your left elbow. Then extend your right arm and lower your right hand to clasp the left hand. This can be very intense, so breathe deeply, and don't force it. Five breaths.

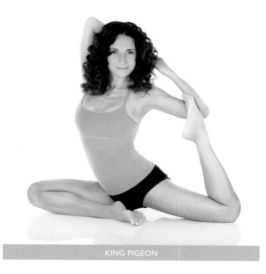

KING PIGEON

## SPLITS

Start by standing on your knees and extend your right leg straight out in front of you so that the heel of your foot is on the floor. Bring both hands to the floor on either side of you. Begin crawling your hands forward as you slowly slide your right foot forward, allowing the back leg to straighten behind you. Stop at the point of intensity, where you can still maintain comfortable breathing. You may need to continue to use your hands to support you on the floor, or you can also prop a bolster or a block underneath your hip. For those of you that can come all the way down, we are selling you to Cirque du Soleil, but before we do, extend both arms overhead, and touch the palms together.

## LOTUS

Begin by sitting on the ground, with your left leg bent in, as if you were sitting cross-legged. Lift your right foot and draw it toward your left groin, resting the top of your right foot on your left thigh. Sit up tall, lengthening through the crown of your head. This may feel very intense for some of you, so if this is your posture today, then great. Stay here and breathe. To move into Lotus, keep your right foot on the top of your left thigh, and draw your left foot out from underneath your right leg. Move mindfully as you bring your left foot to the top of your right thigh. Breathe deeply into any intensity you feel here. If you feel acute pain, release the posture immediately.

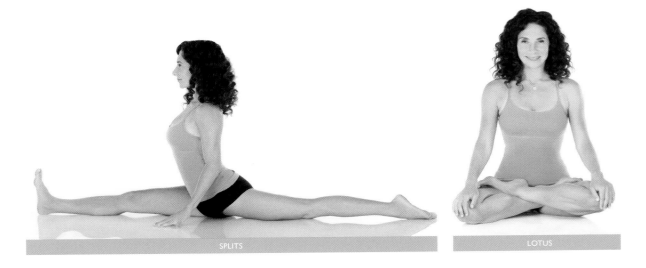

SPLITS          LOTUS

## FROG

Start in tabletop position, with your knees directly under your hips. Keeping your hips and knees in one line, slide your knees away from each other and slowly lower down onto your forearms. Bring your shins perpendicular to the thighs and flex your feet. Draw your navel slightly in toward your spine to maintain length in your lower back and breathe. To deepen the experience, move your knees farther away from each other and lower your torso and arms to the floor. Breathe. Feel your hips and groin muscles opening. Breathe.

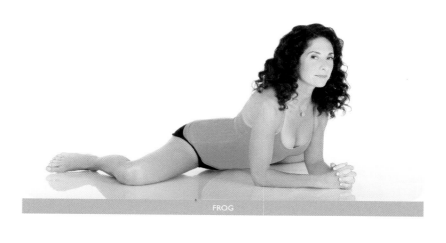

FROG

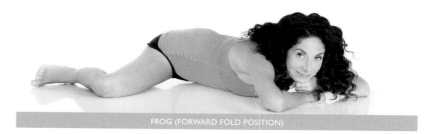

FROG (FORWARD FOLD POSITION)

With your feet hip-width apart, crouch down and place your hands flat on the floor, directly behind your feet. Rest your hips onto your triceps as you slowly begin to shift your weight back, and at the same time press firmly into the floor with your hands. As your feet come up, hook your toes together. Once you get comfortable here and start developing more upper-body strength, you can extend both legs straight. Use your abdominal muscles for strength and stability, and continue to press firmly into the floor until your arms are eventually straight.

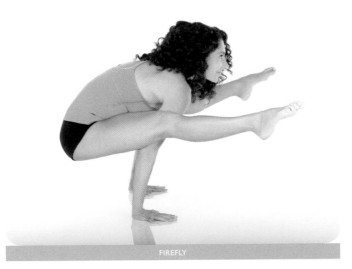

FIREFLY

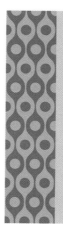

- **JOURNAL**

  "Life is hard, but I am harder." I saw this quote on an author's desk, reminding him to persevere. Find a saying that makes you feel strong.

- **GRATITUDE LIST**

  Make a list that includes some of your most difficult situations.

- **BREATHING EXERCISE**

## *Recipe*: GREEN-HERB OMELET WITH GOAT CHEESE

Breakfast is my favorite meal. Make sure that you remember to feed yourself so that you have the energy for transformation. Here's a recipe from celebrity chef Vikki Krinski.

**5 egg whites**
**½ cup fresh spinach**
**3 tablespoons diced green pepper**
**2 tablespoons freshly chopped dill**
**2 tablespoons chopped chives**
**2 tablespoons fresh goat cheese**
**1 piece toasted gluten-free bread**

Lightly spray pan and heat to medium low. Add egg whites to cover pan. Once solid white, add all the ingredients on one side of omelet. Gently fold other side over and keep on heat for a minute longer to melt cheese. Toast the bread. Spread 1 teaspoon Earth Balance on toast or enjoy dry.

# DAY 17

## MAKE IT SEXY
### *Sex It Up*

I knew the title of this chapter would get your attention—who doesn't love to talk about sex? Here's the deal: Sexual energy is the most potent creative energy you possess. After all, you can create an entire human being with that energy. Now imagine all of that potential channeled toward re-creating your body? Thinking about sex increases the intensity of your workout, helps to get the heart pumping, and has been scientifically proven to cause you to burn more calories when you imagine it. If you don't believe me, don't take my word for it. . . . Try it! This actually works.

*"I'm bringing sexy back."*

— JUSTIN TIMBERLAKE

If you are having trouble getting going with your workout, thinking about someone that you have a crush on is completely motivating. And don't worry, nobody can tell what you're thinking about while you exercise. No one is reading your mind, so it's okay to think of someone other than your partner, although if that's working for you, you have some homework—a make-out session!

Often when I feel myself fading during a workout, I think about a secret crush I have. I may think about a great kiss or even just the feeling of someone's hand on my leg, and it will rev me up. I actually got through my father's passing with a daily shot of espresso and an obsessive crush I had on one of my unsuspecting students. (He never knew, by the way. I could barely look him in the eye or say a word to him, even when he spoke to me.) If you don't already have a crush on someone, go out and get one. If this does not work for you,

159

press play on any Prince track. You don't really need the crush material, because sexual energy exists within you. That's what I'm talking about. Bring the sexy to your workout.

I tend to use the power of sexual energy to fuel me, rather than act on it directly. My feeling is that if I can create an entire being with that energy, if I can use it for whatever I want in my life and transform my sacred body with it, then I'm going to channel it in empowering ways! And frankly, I often find that just being in the presence of someone you are attracted to can ignite the dormant Goddess within.

In my opinion, nothing is sexier than moving your body. You want to get that energy down low. The second chakra, the energy center that is located in the groin/reproductive-system area is related to the water element, the color orange, and pleasure. It is about intimacy, and it is what enables us to relate with others on a very deep level. In astrology, there are two areas of the zodiac that represent sex. One area is regarded as the house of creativity, children, play, and having fun. The other is also connected to other people's money (the currency with which we interrelate with others) and death (as they say in French, orgasm is a "little death"), so we are talking about a level of transcendence that ultimately leads to a catharsis. And it all just started with a silly, little crush.

## ✾ ACTION CHECKLIST

### INTENTION: *Be passionate!*

Hot, hot, hot! It's very sexy to be sweaty and working hard. It's very sexy to be present, self-possessed, and in control of your body. It's incredibly sexy to have power over your thoughts and passions and to direct the energy so that you may manifest what you want for your body.

### PLAYLIST: *Make It Sexy*

When I first started teaching, I realized that most of the songs on my motivating playlists were about sex. Go figure. Try this playlist, but experiment with your own tracks to see what gets you going.

"To Turn You On," Roxy Music

"Sexy Boy," Air

"Do Ya Think I'm Sexy," Rod Stewart

"Sex and Candy," Marcy Playground

"Sexy MF," Prince

"You Sexy Thing," Hot Chocolate

"Sexy Back," Justin Timberlake

"Sex on Fire," Kings Of Leon

"Sexual Healing," Marvin Gaye

### YOGALOSOPHY ROUTINE VARIATION

Think about the greatest make-out session or sexual experience that you have ever had (or wished you'd had). Pretend that you are performing the routine for that person you have the hots for. Wear lingerie during the routine. Add twenty-five to one hundred extra pelvic tucks to the routine, depending on your stamina.

### CARDIO OPTION

Perform a strip tease, have a make-out session, or actual sex (fun fact: the average-size woman burns about 200 calories during a half hour of sex!). If you don't have a partner to do this with, try taking a pole-dancing class, or dance in your living room wearing some sexy lingerie.

# POSE OF THE DAY

This is a yoga trick that will improve your sex life. Do I have your full attention now? If you have been to a yoga class, you may have heard them say it. Mula Bandha. It's an energy "lock," and the way you do it is just like a Kegel exercise. If you don't know what a Kegel exercise is, pretend that you are peeing and then stop the flow, midstream. Then hold that for a few seconds. This energy lock, or mula banda, is a part of certain yoga classes because one way to keep our energy contained is by closing off the openings where energy is lost. We reserve our energy for where it is needed.

No matter how you slice it, this is a great exercise for you, and the best part about it is you can do it any time, anywhere, and no one will know.

Either from a seated or standing position, squeeze the PC muscle (the pubococcygeus muscle, or that sensitive area between your front and rear private parts) and hold for ten counts. Release and repeat. Try doing eight of these between each of the twelve Yogalosophy routine moves.

PHYSICAL BENEFITS: Builds core strength.

HEALING BENEFITS: Increases energy and vitality. Improves concentration and mental clarity.

EMOTIONAL ASPECTS: Grounding. Improves intimacy.

## EXTRA CREDIT: *Invite friends out to a sensual dinner.*

Go out to dinner with someone, or a few people. Order a healthy meal, but the restriction is you can only feed others, and you are not allowed to feed yourself. Others may feed you.

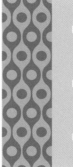

■ **JOURNAL**
Write the sexiest entry you can think of. Let your imagination run wild.

■ **GRATITUDE LIST**
List five things that bring you pleasure.

■ **BREATHING EXERCISE**

## *Recipe:* CHOCOLATE CHIA SEED PUDDING

This sweet and sensual chocolate concoction comes courtesy of culinary expert Melissa Costello, creator of Karma Chow. Beware: According to Melissa, this recipe is known to make you feel irresistible. Indulge and enjoy!

½ cup chia seeds
2 cups almond or coconut milk, unsweetened
½ cup cashews
5 pitted dates
2 tablespoons maple syrup
2-3 tablespoons raw cacao powder (depending on your taste)
1 teaspoon vanilla extract
½ teaspoon cinnamon
Pinch of salt
Fresh berries for garnish (your choice)

Place chia seeds in a medium-sized glass or metal bowl. Blend remaining ingredients together in a high-powered blender until creamy smooth. Pour over chia seeds. Stir well to combine and let sit for about 10-15 minutes or until pudding thickens. Serve room temperature or refrigerate and serve cold. Top with fresh berries. Serves 4.

# DAY 18

## STAY POSITIVE

### *What You Think about Expands*

The saying "What you think about expands" is true, so do yourself a favor: don't focus on how big your butt is! Have you ever noticed that staying positive can be a challenge? It feels as if we're taught that when we speak highly of ourselves, it's boastful, and that it's more appealing to be self-deprecating. False modesty is not true humility, but it is a backdrop for keeping yourself stuck in a state of lack. The ego has just as much invested in you staying small, so that it can search for things "out there" to accomplish and feed it. The more meekly you act, the smaller your world becomes.

> *"When you change the way you look at things, the things you look at changes."*
>
> — WAYNE DYER

Think about it: Have you ever had someone come up to you and say, "Wow, you look great; you look like you've lost weight," and you say, "Nah," and before you know it, the pounds have crept on somehow. Or perhaps you've experienced the flip side of the coin: When you make a decision to really celebrate your body by accepting those few extra pounds and not worrying about your weight, and the pounds suddenly peel off? If you know what I'm talking about, you know it makes no logical sense. At least it doesn't make sense within the limited ways of thinking. I believe that our bodies respond to our acceptance. When we accept ourselves, the negative self-talk dissolves, and the body can fall into its natural state.

With that in mind, consider this: It is your birthright to be happy in the present moment. By focusing on the positive, you will become joyous regardless of whether anything on the outside changes; somehow, everything begins to shift into place. When you focus on the positive, you see the positive and it expands your happiness quotient. When you feel expanded, the world appears to unfold before you to mirror that expansiveness, as if you have a direct line to the secrets of the universe.

When I first started to watch my mind during exercise, I observed the way I spoke to myself. If I started grunting or complaining about the teacher or how hot it was or how sore I felt, it seemed that I would get sluggish and I would want to stop or give up. The same thing happened when I set a really high goal for myself. For example, say I set out to do a really hard three-hour workout to make up for the exercise that I had missed for the last three days. With such an extreme goal ahead of me, I would end up petering out about halfway through, and it would feel like a loss since I didn't live up to my expectations, even though it was a long workout.

Whereas when I would just plan on making it to the gym and start my workout with no pressure, checking in every ten minutes to see if I could go further, I would feel so proud that I had done much more than I had set out to do! In the past, I would focus on where I was not, rather than acknowledging where I was. So focus on the positive today. Think of how much you have already explored and how you just have this day to be happy with, so go for it!

## ⚛ ACTION CHECKLIST

**INTENTION:** *Yes.*

Say YES to everything today. No matter what comes your way, it's a YES.

**PLAYLIST:** *Happy, Joyous, and Free*

"Guidi Diop," Wasis Diop

"Positive Vibrations," Bob Marley

"Positive," Spearhead & Michael Franti

"Jammin'," Bob Marley

"Where Are You Going," Dave Matthews Band

"Ain't Goin' To Goa," Alabama 3

"In My Dreams," Des'ree

"I Know I'm Not Alone," Michael Franti

"Have a Good Time," Simon & Garfunkel

"The Girl from Ipanema," Stan Getz and Astrud Gilberto

## YOGALOSOPHY ROUTINE VARIATION

Add five pliés, five lunges, and five squats to the Yogalosophy routine. This will bring more bounce into your step and more energy to your day. When you bump it up this way, you will receive maximum benefits with very little extra effort.

## CARDIO OPTION

Run for thirty minutes. Get those endorphins kicking in to enhance your mood and boost your energy level.

DAY 18

# POSE OF THE DAY

## PIGEON

Pigeon opens up the hips to make you more receptive. Since you are using your legs to get out there and explore the world, you must take the time to open the hips so that they can become more pliable and you are more available to receive.

Begin in Downward Facing Dog. Raise your right leg up behind you and swing the leg, stepping forward to the midpoint of your hands. Allow your right knee to open out to the right, angling your knee at two o'clock. Your left leg should be extended behind you, internally rotated so that your hips are squared and your knee is facing the floor. If you do not feel the stretch on the outer right glute, you can slide the foot up a little higher. Stay here, or deepen the stretch by placing the forearms on the floor, or extending completely forward and resting your forehead on the ground.

PHYSICAL BENEFITS: Stretches glutes, stretches groin, psoas muscle, and hip flexor. Helps with lower back pain, stretches the back.

HEALING BENEFITS: Brings blood flow to the hip area, stimulating the circulation and energy to move through the joints. Stimulates internal organs.

EMOTIONAL ASPECTS: Helps you develop courage and get unstuck.

MODIFICATIONS: Reclining Pigeon (see page 180.)

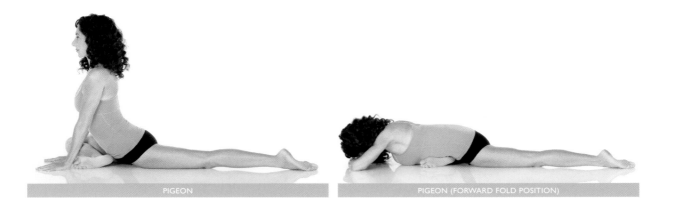

PIGEON                         PIGEON (FORWARD FOLD POSITION)

## EXTRA CREDIT: *Read the masters.*

One of the greatest tools for expanding positivity is reading the words of the masters. Choose teachers that are inspiring to you, and read their writing as inspiration. Reading these words will begin to change your mental outlook and your cells will sing. We are all on the road together, and books like these can serve as maps for us to follow, if they move us or speak to us. Create your map to the final destination.

Here are my tricks for staying positive:

- Read the masters.

- Assume the position of the masters.

- Make a place to honor all aspects of your expanded self.

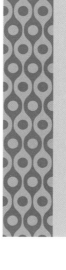

■ **JOURNAL**

At the end of the day, write down all of the things you said "yes" to today, and how that positivity enhanced your life.

■ **GRATITUDE LIST**

Instead of the gratitudes, make a list today of five things you're good at, or things you've done well—physically, personally, on any level. This will keep your motivation high today.

■ **BREATHING EXERCISE**

# Recipe: SOUTHWESTERN VEGAN SALAD

In the spirit of expansion, it is important to explore our flavor palate without expanding our waistlines. This salad it tasty and will work for all diet options.

**2 15-ounce cans black beans, well-drained**
**1½ cups corn**
**1 diced red or yellow bell pepper**
**1 diced avocado (optional)**
**3 chopped tomatoes**
**4 chopped green onions**
**⅓ cup chopped fresh cilantro**
**⅓ cup lime juice**
**⅓ cup olive oil**
**½ teaspoon salt, or to taste**
**⅛ teaspoon cayenne pepper**

Combine the beans, corn, bell pepper, avocado, tomatoes, onion and cilantro in a large mixing bowl and gently toss. Whisk together the remaining ingredients, then pour over the beans mixture and gently stir to combine. Chill one hour before serving.

# DAY 19

## EXPLORE YOUR FREEDOM
### *The Journey Is the Destination*

H ere's some instant enlightenment: There is nothing wrong with you. There is nothing to fix. This old way of thinking, the one that probably got you to pick up the book that "Jennifer Aniston's yoga instructor" wrote, is one that comes from hoping that someone else has the answer, or holds the key, to your fulfillment. I'm here to tell you there is nothing you are lacking; everything you need is already within you, and when you reclaim every facet of who you are, you will understand a new freedom and a new peace. You will come to realize that all is well in your world. It is that sense of wholeness and holistic living that affects the way you feed yourself, your self-expression, and hence your freedom.

> *"I am already given the power that rules my fate. And I cling to nothing, so I will have nothing to defend. I have no thoughts, so I will see. I fear nothing, so I will remember myself. Detached and at ease, I will dart past the Eagle to be free."*
>
> — CARLOS CASTANEDA

There is no freedom without discipline. These two qualities are, in fact, the flip side of the same coin. There's that coin again, which came up in the day about balance. Since the universe is a dance of balance and blending, and yoga is the blending or the marriage of the two energies (and you are the miracle that sits between the two, containing and expressing the energy!), we must have one in order to have the other.

So in a sense, the more you exercise your discipline, the more freedom you will have. The feeling of being free in your body comes from the expansion that you feel once you have built that foundation of strength. Imagine a child who has a very stable home base so that he or she has the confidence to explore beyond their immediate world. Or think of a tree that is able to grow as tall as its roots reach down deep. It is like that with your work, too. If you are disciplined and work consistently, and you somehow manage to stay with your intentions long enough, you will have more options for growth. Perhaps you will make more money so you will be free to travel, take a special class, or enjoy a day off. Of course, you can take a trip without the discipline, but then you may not have the means or you may be dependent on others to take you there, and thus, have less freedom.

It goes like this with the body as well. As you have continued your daily routine, you have developed the strength, flexibility, and the practice to venture out into uncharted territory. There is something in you that is growing and expanding and is joyful. Today, we move past our structure and our limitations to bring together every facet of ourselves that we've worked on thus far. This is a day to travel light and explore.

I understand that the notion of exploration might be intimidating. Early on it was for me too, but through an unfortunate school experience (that turned into a great one), I learned the power of venturing outward. I was always a very shy and timid girl. I would fear that if I dialed the number to hear the automated voice offer the correct time (a quick way to find out the exact time when I was a kid), a real person might answer. I was afraid that if someone live answered, I wouldn't know what to say. My world could have gotten very small. I was a straight-A student in public school and fit in nicely with the other kids, but something was restrictive about fitting in. Even though I worked well within the school system, I was still not fully myself.

In the fourth grade, I had a horrible teacher and my parents decided to pull me out of my grammar school and put me into a new school for experiential learning. It turned out to be a tremendously positive change for me. We went to school in a multicolored van and used the city of Los Angeles as our resource. We took field trips all around Los Angeles, did our academics in libraries, and had lunch in the various parks. The entire student body of about thirty kids had a two-week orientation, and then we were empowered to make the rules of the school ourselves. Each week we were presented with an itinerary of our activities, and each of us would create and sign an agreement sheet that we would present to the teacher, one-on-one, outlining what we were committing to academically. The focus of the school was to develop the whole child. Not just the intellect, but the creative, physical, psychological, and emotional aspects as well. We were encouraged to be 100 percent ourselves. We were given a voice, and we were supported in how to learn, not what to learn. We packed light and explored.

For instance, once we went on a field trip to an architect's office, took notes, and asked questions. Then we were to journal about the experience and turn it in. We followed that up by building a geodesic dome together as a group, then we split off into teams to create a model city. Our cities were influenced by our visits to the gas company or the sewage system during the same week. This expanded and integrated curriculum exposed me to so many options and facets of myself. I became aware of things I likely would never have tried, and I discovered skills and interests I didn't know I possessed.

So today I am encouraging you to take your insides outside. Get out there and try some experiential learning. This earth is a living library, and it is available to you. You don't have to travel to a different country or even another city. Just don't do the same thing the same way again today. Tired of the same old, same old? Well, you have a nice, strong foundation, and I give you permission to find out what you want to learn.

## ❧ ACTION CHECKLIST

**INTENTION:** *Seeker.*

Go on a treasure hunt at a spiritual bookstore. Enter the bookstore and pick up the first purple book you see. Ask a question and open the book to any page. There's your message.

**PLAYLIST:** *Freedom Mix*

Add your own freedom songs, or take the ones you like and leave the rest.

"Spiritual High, Part III," Moodswings

"Freedom," Jurassic 5

"Freedom 90," George Michael

"I Feel Free," Cream

"I'm Free," The Who

"Free Bird," Lynard Skynard

"Everybody's Free (to Wear Sunscreen)," Baz Luhrmann

"Free Xone," Janet Jackson

"Free Fallin'," Tom Petty

"I Will Be Free," Nil Lara

"One Road to Freedom," Ben Harper

**YOGALOSOPHY ROUTINE VARIATION**

Add variations to the daily poses and toners (see instructions below).

- **CALF RAISES:** Keep your heels lifted and lower your hips down in a slow four-count and then back up.
- **CHAIR:** Raise your heels for a four-count.
- **LUNGE:** Add eight reps of a pelvic tilt.
- **PLIÉ SQUATS:** Raise both heels up. Hold.

- **DOWNWARD FACING DOG:** Add a hamstring curl by drawing the heel toward your butt. Eight reps each side.
- **SIDE LEG LIFT:** Straighten your leg out to the side. Flex your foot. Do eight leg lifts.
- **SUPERMAN:** Squeeze your inner thighs and bring your heels and toes together behind you. Pulse for eight reps.
- **PUSH-UPS:** After dips, do one more set with fingers turned in and elbows out to the side, to work your chest.
- **UPWARD FACING DOG:** Press your palms into floor, and lift your thighs off the mat. Look over your right shoulder behind you for a stretch. Switch sides.
- **SIDE PLANK:** Raise your top leg. Hold.
- **PELVIC TUCKS:** Bring hands beneath your shoulders. Press yourself up to Wheel.
- **HEEL TOUCHES:** Bring your feet apart and press your knees together. Do a side reach from heel to heel to work your waist and obliques.
- **V-UPS:** Add twenty crunches, curling your elbows to your knees and your knees into your elbows.

**CARDIO OPTION**

Drive to a new location and take a thirty- to sixty-minute walk. Explore that new location. Or get thee to a treadmill. Walk at an incline, and every four minutes break free by sprinting for one minute. Do this five times.

DAY 19

# POSE OF THE DAY

Time to explore and try a harder pose you may not have had the courage to attempt. Explore it with passion and compassion for your body. Remember where you have come from. You are strong and you can bring that discernment into your attempts as well. I am going to give you one option to try, the very sassy Bird of Paradise.

Start in Warrior 2. Place your right palm to the inside of the right heel. You can press your leg open with your right arm. Extend the left arm straight up, and prepare to wrap. Reach the left arm around your lower back. Wrap your bottom (right) arm underneath your bent (right) leg. Clasp the hands, so that you are wrapping. This may be enough for you. Remember to take things at your own pace. Keep leaning the torso back and pressing the hips forward so that the knee, shoulder, and head are aligned. If you are ready to explore and challenge yourself a little more, look down to the floor, shift the body weight slightly to the front foot, while maintaining the bind, and step your left foot up to meet the right. (This takes me a few steps.) Now transfer the body weight over to the left foot, as you slowly stand up to balance. Find that extension. If you want to go further still, then extend and straighten your right leg. After holding several breaths, bend down as you lower the right foot to the floor and step back. Then open the arms and feel exuberant that you tried the pose, regardless how far you got! Repeat on other side. Pass out.

PHYSICAL BENEFITS: Strengthens legs, stretches inner thighs, groin, shoulders, and chest.

HEALING BENEFITS: Focuses the mind. Good for gracefulness and balance.

EMOTIONAL ASPECTS: Brings emotional balance and calm.

MODIFICATIONS: Just the wrap. Or you can walk the back foot up to the front, but do not stand.

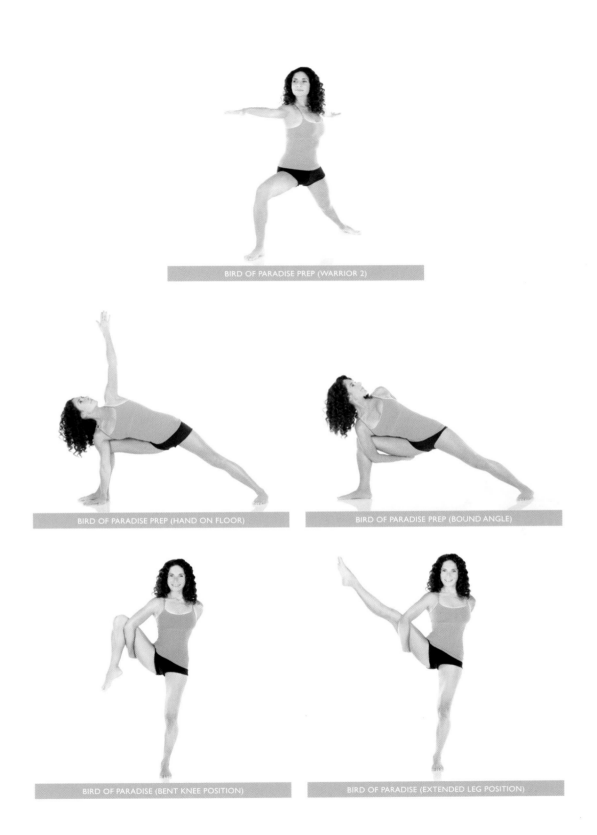

BIRD OF PARADISE PREP (WARRIOR 2)

BIRD OF PARADISE PREP (HAND ON FLOOR)

BIRD OF PARADISE PREP (BOUND ANGLE)

BIRD OF PARADISE (BENT KNEE POSITION)

BIRD OF PARADISE (EXTENDED LEG POSITION)

**EXTRA CREDIT:** *Be a journalist.*

Go somewhere you don't know very well—a place that you are interested in—and ask questions. Explore. Take notes. Write about the experience later. It doesn't have to be the facts, although you can include them if you like.

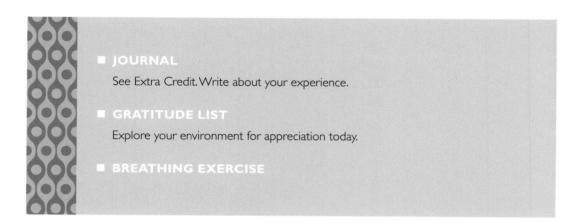

- **JOURNAL**
  See Extra Credit. Write about your experience.

- **GRATITUDE LIST**
  Explore your environment for appreciation today.

- **BREATHING EXERCISE**

*Recipe:* **ERIKA'S SALAD**

Thanks to journalist and adventuring party girl Erika Lenkert for providing this recipe.

**2 tablespoons vegetable oil**
**2 teaspoons champagne vinegar**
**½ teaspoon Dijon mustard**
**¼ teaspoon coarse salt and generous pinch freshly ground pepper**
**6 cups mixed greens**
**1 celery stalk, sliced into ½-inch-wide bites**
**1 tablespoon dried currants or raisins**
**1 tablespoon toasted almond slivers**
**1 cubed red apple**
**1 grilled boneless, skinless chicken breast, baked and torn into bite-size bits**

Mix the oil, vinegar, mustard, salt, and pepper in the bottom of a salad bowl. Throw the rest of the ingredients in the bowl, toss, and serve. Delish!

# DAY 20

## RESPECT YOUR LIMITATIONS
### *Obstacles Are Opportunities*

**Y**ou have built up your strength and stamina and have really been challenging yourself. Today I would like you to pull back and allow your body to recover. If you feel like you are reaching a plateau or hitting a wall, you may need to take a step back and re-evaluate where you are today. If factoring recovery into your process feels like you're slacking off, you're not. I've never gotten into shape any faster by being hard and relentless with myself. This is how an amateur thinks. Sometimes we hit a wall so that we can regroup. Obstacles are opportunities.

*"There is no such thing as a problem without a gift for you in its hands."*

— RICHARD BACH

What if everything in your life is exactly as it should be? What if the things that are seemingly holding you back today are actually there to teach you how to develop the skills to better manifest your dreams? Obstacles are opportunities in disguise. In order to grow and expand, it's necessary to respect discipline and structure. Certain laws of structure bind us all. For instance, your body has a physical structure. Some people are able to press their heels into the mat in Downward Facing Dog, while others struggle to touch their toes in a Forward Bend.

Each of us has limitations to respect and to work with. That does not mean you cannot do a Standing Forward Bend, but you may need to modify by bending your knees. You may become more flexible and have less aches and pains; in fact, you most likely will, but the only reason to have such a goal is to provide space for growth. Regardless of your talents, at some point, you will hit your limit. A key to developing skillfulness is identifying strengths and weaknesses, understanding how to work within your own constraints, as well as knowing when to push through the habitual patterns that hold you back.

The most satisfying and gratifying accomplishments are experienced as a result of hard work, perseverance, and seeing obstacles as opportunities. I know this firsthand. I would never have dreamed that an injury, which left me flat on my back, would allow me the time and patience to develop a business skill, or give me the compassion for a student who has difficulty stepping into a lunge. It was my back injury that allowed me the opportunity to be where I am today, with the skill set that I have. It's like that saying: I pray for patience, and God gives me long lines.

At this phase, I would like you to ruminate over what is working for you, which of your limitations must be respected, and whether it's appropriate for you to push at this time. Bringing maturity, authority, and structure to your practice is the most responsible and useful skill in attaining your long-term goal, which is only one week away! You can see the top of the mountain and the finish line. The amateur may become overly excited or impatient, but the master stays steady here, and in fact pulls back to ruminate over the past and ponder the future, creating a map of the terrain that can be navigated through the home stretch.

Since we are paring down in preparation, there is no rush as we walk through this energetic doorway. A new week, and yes . . . a new you! Who knows what you may find. Do not rush toward your goals and resolutions immediately, but use this opportunity to set yourself up for success.

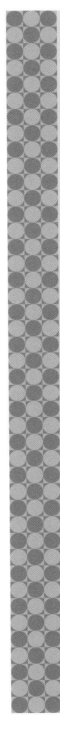

## ❧ ACTION CHECKLIST

**INTENTION:** *Maturity.*

Respect your limitations. When you are this close to your goal, it is hard to pull back. It takes a lot of maturity and self-respect to acknowledge where you truly are.

**PLAYLIST:** *Mellow Mix*

Play your favorite mellow music—something that supports you. I find that as I mature, I mellow. Here's a mix I really like. I made it when I was a little low.

"Night Bird," Deep Forest

"Everloving," Moby

"Teardrop," Massive Attack

"The Glass Bead Game," Thievery Corporation

"#41," Dave Matthews Band

"Tarana," Thievery Corporation

"Slow Marimbas," Peter Gabriel

"Distractions," Zero 7

"I Still Care for You," Ray Lamontagne

"Higher Ground," Weekend Players

"Even after All," Finley Quay

"Lover Lay Down," Dave Matthews Band

"Tear of the Moon," Coyote Oldman

## YOGALOSOPHY ROUTINE VARIATION

Regroup and address whatever area of your body is bothering you. Knees hurt? Lower back sore? See today's four different restorative poses to help you recover.

## CARDIO OPTION

Drop the routine and go for a leisurely twenty to sixty-minute walk today. It's time to evaluate what is working for you and where you need a tune-up. You must climb your own mountain now. Use your walk to review what you have accomplished in the past three weeks and where you aim to go in the final home stretch. During this time, you can create a deliberate terrain for yourself that you can navigate. Eliminate the obsolete and hone in on the beneficial.

DAY 20

# POSES OF THE DAY

## Restorative Poses

Restorative yoga poses will help you to relax the body and go within, while providing an opportunity to renew and heal. Your body actually gets stronger when you are resting. Active exercises break down the muscles and this is your body's time to repair, so passive poses are productive!

### RECLINING PIGEON

Props: Eye pillow, pillow, or hand towel.

Recline on your back. If your head does not rest comfortably on the floor, place a rolled up towel underneath your head. Bend your legs and place the soles of your feet on the floor. Cross your right ankle over your left knee. Flex your right foot. Draw the left knee to your chest and thread your hands, like you're threading a needle, around the left hamstring. Feel the stretch on your outer right hip. Take five to ten deep breaths and repeat on the other side.

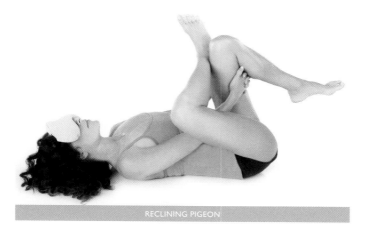

RECLINING PIGEON

### LEGS UP THE WALL

Props: Blankets or bolster. Eye pillow or hand towel.

Fold two blankets so you have a six-inch-high soft support for your lower back. (Or use a bolster.) Place them parallel to and a few inches away from the wall. Hug your knees into your chest, lie on your left side, and then roll onto your right hip, using your left arm to support you as you swing your legs up the wall. You should be supported by the six-inch-thick blankets or bolster from the top of your tailbone to your mid back (shoulder blades can be on floor). Climb your legs up the wall for support. Place an eye pillow or folded hand towel over your eyes and rest here from five to twenty minutes. Breathe into your lower belly, allowing it to relax and expand on the inhale and fall back on the exhale.

### WIDE-LEGGED STANDING FORWARD BEND

Props: Chair

Stand with your legs several feet apart, facing the chair. Make sure your weight is evenly distributed and that the feet are parallel. Hinge at your hips, with a flat back, and bend forward at the hips. Place your hands on the chair. Rest your forehead on the chair. (Option: Use a table or place hands on wall in an "L" shape.)

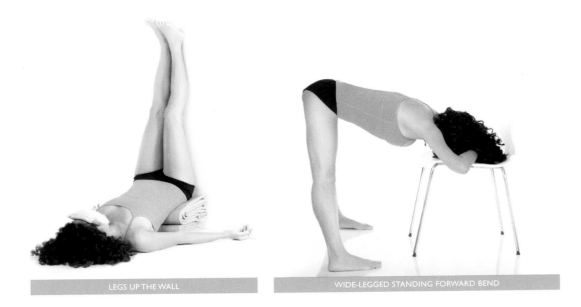

LEGS UP THE WALL · WIDE-LEGGED STANDING FORWARD BEND

# EXTRA CREDIT: *Tips for respecting your limitations.*

## POSTURE MODIFICATIONS

CHILD'S POSE: Hurts your knees? Place a rolled-up towel behind the back of the knees.

DOWNWARD FACING DOG: Hamstrings tight? Bend your knees and/or widen your stance.

Back injury? Place your hands on wall to make an "L" shape with your body. Forward flexion can be harmful when injured.

PLANK POSE: Sway back? Place knees on the floor.

Hurts your wrists? Stand on your fists instead.

TRIANGLE POSE: Cannot bring hand to the floor? Hold your shin, or use a yoga brick or chair.

CAMEL POSE: Not ready to reach the heels? Keep your hands on your hips.

## CONTRAINDICATIONS

Back injuries? Anything lying on your back is safe because the floor is supporting and aligning your spine. Avoid twists.

Twists are NOT appropriate for pregnant women.

## OTHER TIPS

TROUBLE SLEEPING: Try Legs up the Wall.

TIGHT KNEES: Open up with Reclining Pigeon.

BACK IS SEIZED UP: The front of the body may be tightening. Try stretching the hips with a lunge.

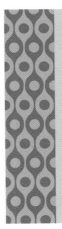

■ **JOURNAL**

Write about a time when you had a setback, and recall the benefits of that time.

■ **GRATITUDE LIST**

Be grateful for your list of obstacles! Yup, put the most difficult at the top of that gratitude list.

■ **BREATHING EXERCISE**

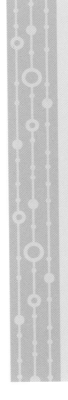

## *Recipe:* HEALING KABOCHA SQUASH AND SAGE BUTTER QUINOA

Sometimes we need a little comfort. When I have injuries, it usually means I need to ground. Enjoy this grounding dish.

½ a medium kabocha squash
3 tablespoons melted coconut oil
½ cup quinoa (prepared per package instructions)
½ tablespoon chopped fresh sage
1 tablespoon minced shallots
½ teaspoon salt

Preheat oven to 400°F. Cut squash in half, scoop out seeds. Use 1 tablespoon coconut oil to coat cut surface of squash. Place cut side down on baking sheet. Bake for 45 minutes. Cool, peel, and cut into 1-inch chunks. Prepare quinoa according to package. Use a food processor to blend coconut oil, sage, shallots, and salt until smooth. Heat mixture in a large pan on low heat for 1 minute. Add quinoa, and stir to combine for 1 minute. Remove from heat and fold in squash.

# DAY 21

## COMMIT TO YOUR GOALS/SELF-MASTERY

### *You've Come This Far. It's Too Late to Quit!*

I have studied with many great teachers, in a lot of different disciplines, but I really didn't enter into mastery until I, myself, became a teacher. That's when I had to began taking inventory of myself and making decisions based on my own inner sense of what I needed. Now it's your turn to become a master of your own program. You are the authority on your own body, so what does it need today?

You are about to start your fourth and final week of the Y28 Revolution. You now have enough self-mastery under your belt to begin to see the results of your hard work. It is very common to start to celebrate prematurely and reward yourself for a job well done by going off course. This is when discipline comes back to the forefront. Goals are reached one step at a time, and seeing your goal through to completion is a pivotal part of the process.

> *"Our deepest fear is not that we are inadequate. Our deepest fear is that we are powerful beyond measure. It is our light, not our darkness that most frightens us. We ask, ourselves 'Who am I to be brilliant, gorgeous, talented, and fabulous?' Actually, who are you not to be?"*
>
> — MARIANNE WILLIAMSON

Obstacles tend to present themselves at this time: the vacation you forgot you scheduled, your child's birthday party where you just have to eat the cake, an injury that you have either pushed through instead of listening to, or a myriad other unique situations and unusual circumstances. So as you recommit to your goal, recall your original intention and look at all that you have accomplished. Know that what you face is simply a common reaction to progress and another reminder to fully commit to YOU.

I remember when I made a decision for myself that I was going to get healthy and lose weight. This was post weight-gain, assault, and self-acceptance. I was out with one of my girlfriends, and we were having breakfast and a smoke. That's right. I went through a smoking phase in my early twenties that was short, but it was a full-blown pack-a-day habit. I used to say that if I could have smoked during sit-ups in an exercise class, I would have. Anyway, we were in the ladies' room, applying mandatory red lipstick, and I said to her, "Would you still be friends with me if I lost weight?" Of course she laughed it off and said yes. We were twenty-four.

Even I was surprised to hear this come out of my own mouth, but apparently there was a part of me that felt my friends were very comfortable with me staying exactly where I was, or rather, I was afraid that people would not like me if I started to shine. If I took care of myself, would other people still care about of me? Would they be there for me emotionally? Would they talk about me behind my back? I cared way too much what everybody else was thinking of me, and my imaginary thoughts were keeping me in limbo-land. At a certain point, I had to let go of what other people thought about my choices and take responsibility for my own actions by focusing on my own needs and committing fully to choices that were self-supporting. Self-mastery has since been a primary theme in my life.

There is a point during your personal revolution when you must break away and be your own authority. For instance, in yoga there are so many philosophies and schools of thought, but which one is the "right" yoga?

Many times, students in a class will wonder if they are practicing "correctly." What is the "right" way to do a pose? What is the "real" yoga? When I hear a teacher claim there is only one right way to do anything, I get suspicious. I am way too rebellious to follow along simply because someone tells me to. Have you noticed that different body types look unalike in the very same pose? I cannot tell you how many times I have been injured because an instructor kept urging me to move into the "correct" position, occasionally placing me in the pose, assuming that my body was ready to go there. No matter how much experience your teacher has, it is essential to be confident in your own body's wisdom. You're the only expert on you.

Almost everything that I truly know and understand has come through experience. No one person can tell me exactly what is right for me, but they can provide me with some guidelines, and once I have moved through it on my own, I am on my way to self-mastery.

We are not here to serve yoga or the tradition of yoga. At least I am not. Yes, there are some people whose life work is dedicated to that, and who are meant to maintain the integrity of the yogic tradition, but that is not what Yogalosophy is about. You are choosing yoga now because you know you want to try it. This is an expression of you. Not something you are squeezing yourself into, like a dress that's two sizes too small. Yoga has become accessible enough for you to claim it—jump in the water and see how yoga can serve you.

Today I want you to "know that you know." Become your own authority on your body. Trust the intention you set for yourself and see it all the way through. Become a master of your own journey.

## ✕ ACTION CHECKLIST

### INTENTION: *I know that I know.*

You know your body better than any teacher. You know the difference between a good hurt and a pain that is a warning signal. It's time to take back the authority over your own body today. I realize it seems easier to turn this over to an expert, but asking someone to sense what is correct for your body structure is like asking an actor to feel your emotions for you. Don't lease your life out to anyone else. Take the wheel and start driving the car to your destination.

### PLAYLIST: *It's All You*

Yup. You thought right. You know best what is most motivating for you. Choose the music that will click with you.

### YOGALOSOPHY ROUTINE VARIATION

It's up to you; just make sure you do some kind of movement for thirty minutes. Make up your own routine based on the moves you have learned and now know.

### CARDIO OPTION

I suggest you structure your workout by planning it out first. Sit and think for yourself before you start. It is intuitive, but give yourself a blueprint, as if you were building a home. This is how I create routines and classes. I intuit the theme, and then I find postures, exercises, and activities that translate the theme through the physical body. I embody the theme. Try it. I know you can do it. You know what is best.

DAY 21

## POSES OF THE DAY

Choose your own from the poses you've learned to date, or refer to B. K. S. Iyengar's book *Light On Yoga* for additional poses.

PHYSICAL BENEFITS: Look it up!

HEALING BENEFITS: Becomming your own best teacher.

EMOTIONAL ASPECTS: Confidence and independence.

## EXTRA CREDIT: *Free choice!*

Pick your own bonus activity today. You know what you enjoy, and how to treat yourself. Maybe it's stealing away for an hour to read a book at a café or taking yourself to a movie. Perhaps it's indulging in a much-deserved massage or a bubble bath. Whatever it is, keep it healthy and all about you.

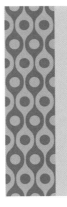

■ **JOURNAL**

■ **GRATITUDE LIST**

Go over the last few weeks and list what you are grateful for that has occurred as a result of your commitment to your goals.

■ **BREATHING EXERCISE**

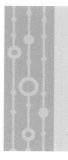

## Recipe: MAKE YOUR OWN.

Create a dish without a cookbook. What do you need that is nourishing? How inventive and resourceful can you be? Get creative!

# DAY 22

## BREAK THE RULES

### *Think for Yourself*

O ften what begins as something unpopular becomes a trend. Personally, I typically rebel against the norm. Perhaps this is because my parents set the example for me to think for myself without worrying about what everybody else was doing. My dad was practicing yoga and eating macrobiotically before anyone in our circle knew what that was.

When we became macrobiotic back in the mid '70s, my parents invited many of their friends over to share the amazing five-course meals my mother made without any meat, dairy, or sugar. Their friends were shocked. If you can't eat butter and meat, then what DO you eat? In fact, my parents lost a lot of friends back in the day because food is social, and it just wasn't acceptable when my dad showed up to lunch dates or parties with his own containers of brown rice, miso soup, and root veggies with seaweed.

> *"What each must seek in his life never was on land or sea. It is something out of his own unique potentiality for experience, something that has never been and never could have been experienced by someone else."*
>
> — JOSEPH CAMPBELL

My mother was so adept at cooking that she would regularly make tempura and millet croquettes. The meals and combinations were endless, often including things like hijiki (seaweed) with burdock (a delicious root vegetable that is very grounding and healing). The crowning glory of the meals was a raw veggie salad, which sounds normal, except for the fact that the water had to be extracted. It was called "pressed salad." It was literally pressed of all liquid. Mom would chop Chinese cabbage, carrots, etc., and then place it all in a stainless steel bowl, with a plate on top of the mixture, and a large rock on top of the plate. Our guests would get a behind-the-scenes look at what appeared to be a medieval ritual. For society in 1977, this was totally weird . . . even in Los Angeles.

My father had no shame. If he felt the need to do a handstand while filling up the car at a gas station, he did it. Can you imagine being an eleven-year-old girl, and your father is actually breaking into a handstand at the pump? Maybe today you might see something like that, but yoga in the 1970s just wasn't cool. There was no such thing as designer workout clothes from Lululemon—it was men wearing "diapers." In fact, the trendy, even mainstream yoga community that you know today did not even exist back then. It needed guys like my dad, who did not care what onlookers or even his friends thought, to break the rules and turn the world upside down. He literally turned upside down daily and changed his perspective.

Growing up in a home like I did, it's easy to see why my journey in finding my individuality began pretty early. Thinking for myself and acting outside the norm became my standard. I left my household and started making money at age fourteen. I didn't have a boyfriend until I was thirty. And at age forty-five, I don't have children or a husband. I invented my own word and coined the term Yogalosophy. I don't even fit in to the yoga community because I am not devotional, nor am I an ass-kicking superhero fitness trainer. I have never even run a triathlon; I just had to risk being me. That's all I can do and be. And the same goes for all of us.

In order to be a trendsetter, the need to be liked has pretty much got to be bulldozed by the demand for invention and the celebration of the individual within the society. All of our great thinkers were considered nuts before the scales tipped in their direction, even at the risk of losing it all. I urge you to think from a place of invention, even if it's just for this day. Who knows, you just might enjoy thinking differently. (Ahem. WHAT box?)

## ❧ ACTION CHECKLIST

### INTENTION: *Intention of invention!*

You have a special spot in the world. Your vantage point is like no other. It's time to break the rules and dare to be yourself. The unique individual that you are is here, and unless you experiment and do it your way, the entire world may miss out on something very valuable that you have to share. You know the saying, if you do the same thing the same way, then nothing is going to change. Well I want you to take that to heart today. Risk being yourself. You just might set a trend.

### PLAYLIST: *Rebel Mix*

Freaks, rebels, and oddballs unite!

"Rebel Rebel," David Bowie

"A Different Drum," Peter Gabriel

"Earthquake Weather," Beck

"Upside Down," Jack Johnson

"Dramastically Different," Beastie Boys

"If He Tries Anything," Ani DiFranco

"Get Ur Freak On," Missy Elliott

"Beautiful Freak," Eels

"Freaky Hijiki," Beastie Boys

### YOGALOSOPHY ROUTINE VARIATION

The Yogalosophy routine you've been doing for the last three weeks was born out of invention. Changing traditional yoga to include toners is something that I thought was crazy at first, but I personally like it and find it effective. I then decided to share it with my clients, and then with the public. I also incorporate some of the cyclical patterns found in astrology, psychology, shamanism, acting, and a variety of philosophies.

Come up with your own routine today, or at least one or two Yogalosophy hybrid moves (a posture/toner combo).

### CARDIO OPTION

Do some activity you've never done before; just make sure to do it for thirty minutes.

- Go mountain climbing.
- Choose a new type of yoga class.
- Go walking or running in a new neighborhood.
- Wake up ridiculously early and work out before sunrise.

Break your own rules.

DAY 22

## POSE OF THE DAY

Make one up. I am not kidding. The Yogalsophy hybrid routine that you have been practicing each day was created out of the spirit of invention. You can try creating a hybrid with one of the poses of the day in this book. Imagine what toning exercise would blend with your favorite pose. Go ahead and try. See, you are gaining independence!

PHYSICAL BENEFITS: Try labeling what you are physically working.

HEALING BENEFITS: Exercises the creator and the inventor. Stretches your mind.

EMOTIONAL ASPECTS: Self-expression, individuality.

## EXTRA CREDIT: *Sing loud and exuberantly.*

Find your favorite album, perhaps even one from childhood, that you used to love to sing along to; music that filled you with emotion—just express yourself openly, freely, and with fierce exuberance. And remember, anyone can sing. You don't have to have a Grammy-worthy voice to belt it out like you mean it!

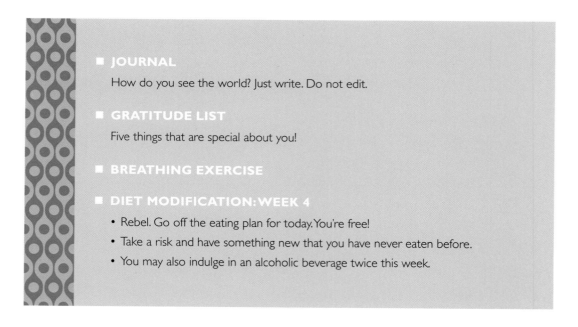

■ **JOURNAL**
How do you see the world? Just write. Do not edit.

■ **GRATITUDE LIST**
Five things that are special about you!

■ **BREATHING EXERCISE**

■ **DIET MODIFICATION: WEEK 4**
- Rebel. Go off the eating plan for today. You're free!
- Take a risk and have something new that you have never eaten before.
- You may also indulge in an alcoholic beverage twice this week.

# Recipe: KANTEN!

When I was a child and we became macrobiotic, there were so many foreign foods. My favorite was kanten. This dessert also called for "agar-agar," which are flakes derived from seaweed, so it is high in iodine. It is used like gelatin (but not made of animal hooves!). Kanten can be made with any combination of fruit juice and fruit. It is chilled in the refrigerator, where it turns into something like jello. To make it creamy like a custard, add kuzu, which is a natural thickener.

**½ cup thinly sliced strawberries**
**½ cup sliced peaches (or any fruit you love)**
**2 cups apple juice**
**2 tablespoons agar-agar flakes (available in Japanese section of many markets)**

Place fruit in a heatproof glass dish or bowl. Mix juice, agar-agar, and salt in a saucepan and bring to a mild boil. Stir until agar-agar is dissolved (about 5 min). Pour over fruit and refrigerate 1 to 2 hours or until firm. Sugarless, packed with sea veggie nutrients, and fun.

# DAY 23

## CHANGE YOUR POINT OF VIEW
### Turn Your Mind Upside Down

We have already established that routine is necessary and that the body thrives on habitual self-care. Yet routine can also mire us in unconscious patterns that put us on autopilot, causing us to miss being present in the moment. So today do it differently. There's nothing like taking an alternate route to work, sitting in another chair on the opposite end of the room, or working out in a different place to wake you up. On a larger scale, by taking on a new perspective you can come to understand opposing points of view, and open your mind to more options for growth and a new approach to old problems.

> "You must be the change you wish to see in the world."
> — MAHATMA GANDHI

I have this thing that I do when I can't conceive of why somebody has a certain behavior: I embody the behavior myself so that I can understand the other person's point of view. This practice began when I was a child and carried over into my career as a young actress. To play a role, you must understand the perspective of the character and find their "truth" and what makes them tick.

When I was in the fifth grade, we had a summer program in my mobile school called Theater on Wheels. We would create spoofs of popular movies and then travel to libraries and convalescent homes to perform for children and the elderly. This one particular summer the Star Wars sequel *The Empire Strikes Back* was very popular. Our spoof was called "The Umpire Strikes Out."

As we were being cast in our roles, I was devastated to see that two of my best girlfriends were cast opposite each other as the popular Ham Salad and Princess Frito Lay. These two girls were pretty and popular, and were the mainstream leads. I was horrified to be cast as Death Vapor, the villain who would kill people with his bad breath. I really hated that I had to find a way to embody this character, and I struggled with my twelve-year-old self for days and days, feeling the feelings that I'm sure my character felt, of being left out and misunderstood.

After I sat with those feelings long enough, I started exploring them and this character. And guess what happened. I started to really enjoy playing the part and coming from this perspective. When I entered as the villain for my solo performance, singing to the tune of "When Will I Be Loved" by Linda Ronstadt, I was greeted with boos and hisses. I ate it up as fuel, and my role ended up being the most celebrated and coveted in the show.

In what way can you embody a different perspective of your very same situation? We each have a role that we play in life. You are not a victim of circumstance, but an active participant. Perhaps you are taking on a new role in life, or there is a way to come to the one you are already playing from a totally new angle. It's up to you to define it and play with it. You are now nearing the end of the program, and you will have a new perspective on what you are capable of. Change your mind and you will change your life and your body.

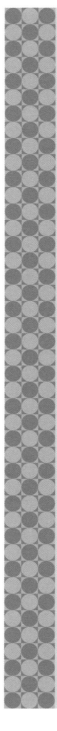

## ✹ ACTION CHECKLIST

**INTENTION:** *Upside down.*

Observe your practice. Be like a scientist. As we've show, the observer changes the outcome of the experiment. The observer is an actual participant. Detach and imagine that you are an experiment. Your practice is an experiment. Once you begin to watch, you will see that your results are much better. Is it your mind changing your body or your body changing your mind?

**PLAYLIST:** *Remixed Covers*

I love the idea of the remix. I love that artists can take a song and create something entirely new with it by placing a different spin on it. Here is a remix playlist for you to enjoy, but feel free to make your own mix.

"Bodyrock," Moby (Rae & Christian Remix)

"Human Nature," Madonna (Howie Tee Remix)

"Gettin' In the Way," Jill Scott (MJ Cole Remix)

"Love Is Stronger Than Pride," Sade (Mad Professor Remix)

"I Want You Back," Jackson 5 (Z-Trip Remix)

"Signed, Sealed, Delivered (I'm Yours)," Stevie Wonder (DJ Smash Essential Funk Mix)

"Papa Was a Rolling Stone," Temptations (DJ Jazzy Jeff Mix)

"Maria Maria," Santana (Wyclef Remix)

"Aquarius," Common (Come Close Remix)

### YOGALOSOPHY ROUTINE VARIATION

Start from the last pose and work your way back to the first. Begin with your left side instead of your right.

### CARDIO OPTION

Today, try pedaling your legs backward on an elliptical trainer or walking backward on a treadmill machine for thirty minutes. In other words, do the opposite of what your body is used to doing. This will work different muscles, and more importantly, it will wake up your mind.

DAY 23

# POSES OF THE DAY

## Inversion Poses

If you are up for a challenge, try a handstand. If not, try a deep Forward Bend. They say that going upside down is the fountain of youth; it reverses the blood flow, which has an antiaging effect. Inversions include Headstand, Handstand, Forward Bend, Dolphin Pose, Wide-legged Forward Bend, and Shoulder Stand.

### PLOUGH

Lie on your back and use your abs to lift the legs over the head until your toes touch the floor; if your toes cannot touch, you can use a wall and place the feet on the wall up over head. Keep your hands on your back, or interlace the fingers and clasp hands to straighten your arms to the floor. Wriggle up on to your shoulders. Hold for five breaths and if you are coming down, roll down one vertabra at a time.

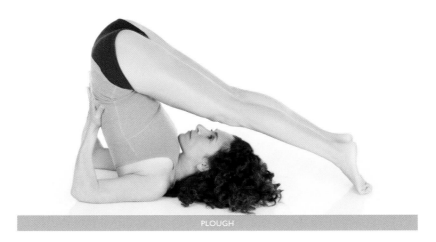

PLOUGH

## SHOULDER STAND

Keeping the elbows shoulder-width apart, bend the elbows and place your hands on your back for support, if they're not there already. One leg at a time, lift the legs. Keep Mountain pose in mind, scooping the tailbone under to keep the spine straight. Press the hips forward and bring the feet back, keeping the legs straight, in one line. Keep hips over shoulders and feet over hips. Work your hands as high up to your shoulders as you can. After five to ten breaths, slowly lower your knees down by your ears, and come out of the pose with control, one vertabra at a time. When your sacrum hits the mat, hug your knees into your chest and gently rock from side to side, releasing your lower back.

PHYSICAL BENEFITS: Stretches every muscle along the back of the body. Helps with sore throat, headaches, sinuses, and varicose veins.

HEALING BENEFITS: Improves circulation, calms thyroid.

EMOTIONAL ASPECTS: Inversions are meant to be the Fountain of Youth. That makes most people feel delighted.

MODIFICATIONS: Do not do if you are on your menstrual cycle. Instead, do Legs Up the Wall (see page 181).

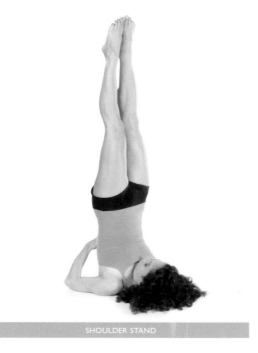

SHOULDER STAND

## EXTRA CREDIT: *Do things differently.*

- Take a different route to work.

- Call someone you have never reached out to before.

- Say hello to a stranger.

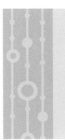

■ **JOURNAL**
Do your morning writing at night.

■ **GRATITUDE LIST**
See if you can come up with five things that you once wanted to change about yourself, but now you accept, love, or embrace. For instance, I used to dislike my curly hair because I could never tame it. But now I love it for its wild exuberance because it feels like an extension of my own nonconformist sensibilities.

■ **BREATHING EXERCISE**

*Recipe:*

Eat breakfast for dinner.

# DAY 24

## BE COMMUNITY-MINDED

### *Join and Be an Activist*

I am not a joiner by nature. I always seem to be the standout, or to have a different opinion that leaves me feeling that I stick out like a sore thumb. It is probably this awkward feeling that has kept me an outsider, turning my energy inward. What I have learned is that group participation is actually the key to harmony. There is a power in the collective energy of a group that creates the trends as well as the revolutions in our society. Since each of us has a specific perspective, we must add to the group by joining and participating. Otherwise, we deny the world our special gifts!

Once I came to own the fact that I was a group leader, I realized that the energy I had been using to self-destruct, when turned in the opposite direction, could power an entire room filled with people. It is my duty to contribute exactly who I am: no more and no less. I felt vulnerable sharing my personal experience as a means to help others. Now I love that it brings me closer to others in my sameness, and that our differences are actually the glue that binds us all together. It can get sticky and messy to share what is personal, yet it also connects us more intimately and opens up opportunities for others to share themselves. This is quite obvious when I am facing a group of students head-on. I get a lot of joy from witnessing the collective moving together, regardless of the seeming differences.

> *"Don't fight forces, use them."*
> — BUCKMINSTER FULLER

When you are in a group class, you are giving energy just by being present! In participating with people you have never met, there is an invisible bond that you have with the teacher right up front and the person in the way back, left side of the room that strengthens everyone. I have taken this experience a step further by using it to give back to the community, teaching classes for group charities. This added another lovely dimension of connection, and it enhanced the collective energy as we extended beyond the classroom and into the world. There is a deep sense of gratitude mixed with the humility of giving that fosters an environment of appreciation, goodwill, and community. What we consciously create together, particularly in the service of good, can be magical.

I feel this is an amazing time to get clearer on our dreams, and to begin living in a way that is in alignment with community. This is especially true given the shifting climate of our economy, where people are turning to each other for support. It doesn't take much to be part of the greater good. Whether it's joining a communal garden where you plant affordable organic produce, mentoring a child that needs assistance, launching a recycling initiative, or organizing a group walk to pick up trash on the beach, there is always something that you can do to help out in your community. Joining together to take action and make the world a little better is a self-esteem builder. The beauty of reaching out is that no matter if you are on the giving or receiving end, it is the connection that matters. The idea that each of us matters is the attitude shift that will bring change and help us to reshape our world directly.

The options for activism and community engagement are endless. Every gesture, big or small, adds to the collective outcome. Your positive energy will have an impact! So this is the day to get your hands dirty and your feet wet. Dare to get involved. Recognize that your actions will not only help others, but it will also bond you more deeply with your community.

## ✖ ACTION CHECKLIST

### INTENTION: *One among many.*

There is power in the group. Remember: It's the collective that creates the trends of society as well as the revolutions. We invent our world together, cocreating and sharing ideas and energies. Even within a group, each of us is a unique individual adding our own personal energy, and each of us has a perspective that no one else has. We each experience the exact same event from a slightly different angle. That is why it is your job to contribute exactly who you are.

### PLAYLIST: *One Among Many*

This playlist is made up of bands with a breakout front man (or woman).

"Bad," U2

"Brass in Pocket," Pretenders

"Independent Women," Destiny's Child

"Seven Nation Army," The White Stripes

"Shake It Out," Florence and the Machine

"Ants Marching," Dave Matthews Band

"Wrapped Around Your Finger," The Police

"Crawing Back to You," Tom Petty

"Never Can Say Goodbye," Jackson 5

### YOGALOSOPHY ROUTINE VARIATION

Take a group yoga class instead of your private routine. You know that class in your community? It's time to take the risk and be among others who are taking care of themselves just the way you want to take care of yourself. You are ready. You can be exactly you. Notice how that group inspires you. You may be inspiring the person right beside you, just by showing up.

### CARDIO OPTION

Try a local group cardio class of any kind. Feel your place in the room, and know that you are directly helping the people in the room. You are actually feeding off of their energy and they are feeding off of yours.

DAY 24

## POSE OF THE DAY

Try a new pose in class today!

PHYSICAL BENEFITS: Ask your teacher about the new pose.

HEALING BENEFITS: See above.

EMOTIONAL ASPECTS: Notice the effect on you. Declare it.

MODIFICATIONS: If you need to tone it down, ask the teacher, or allow your body to help you find the modification. Be mindful.

## EXTRA CREDIT: *Be one among the many.*

The extra credit can either be leading a group of friends through a class, or attending or putting together a group class for your favorite charity. And if you can get a group hug going, consider that fifty extra credit points.

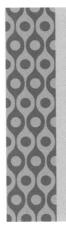

■ **JOURNAL**
Write about a cause that means something to you. Can you plan something that makes you an activist?

■ **GRATITUDE LIST**
Make this gratitude list about your community and your friendships.

■ **BREATHING EXERCISE**

# *Recipe:* JULIE MORGAN'S ARTICHOKE DIP

Julie Morgan is an amazing make-up artist and part of the beauty team that surrounds Ricki Lake and chef Giada de Laurentiis. She's a team player who makes things happen, including delicious recipes, so I always look forward to being invited to a potluck dinner or party where Julie will be.

**2 cups fresh artichoke hearts, cleaned and cooked**
**1 can cannellini beans, drained and rinsed**
**½ cup tahini**
**2 garlic cloves, minced**
**juice of 2 lemons**
**2 teaspoons ground cumin**
**1 teaspoon sea salt**
**⅓ cup extra-virgin olive oil**

Add artichokes, cannellini beans, tahini, garlic, lemon juice, cumin, and salt to the bowl of a food processor; blend together, adding olive oil in a slow steady stream until smooth. Add warm water to reach desired consistency. Add more lemon juice and salt if needed.

# DAY 25

## MEDITATE

### *Create a Spirit Ritual*

E ven for a yoga instructor, meditation can be a challenge. When I find myself busy, I make excuses like, "yoga is my moving meditation," and while it is, only I truly know when I am making that contact, when I am creating a sacred space for my personal connection to inspiration. What if I stay still? What may arise from within me? What may be delivered to my front door? I remember when I was a child, someone said to me, "When you are lost, stay where you are. You will be found." I spend so much time racing around. I just may be outrunning a spirit that is trying to make a connection with me. When I've felt lost in my own life, my connection to stillness in meditation has been profound. If I want spirit to find me, I must sit still.

*"Let the water settle; you will see the moon and stars mirrored in your being."*

— RUMI

Yogi masters say that meditation is the true yoga, and that the real purpose of the physical practice—twisting, contorting, and exhausting ourselves—is so we can ultimately sit still with mindful breathing. Easier said than done, right? My "monkey mind" is racing ninety miles a minute with planning my grocery list, thoughts about my future, and reruns of my life from this morning or even twenty years ago. It seems nearly impossible to stop the endless whirl.

Most of our thoughts tend to be repetitive and can be categorized as follows: worrying about the past, planning for the future, listing, and judging. A very basic form of meditation is to notice what type of thinking you are doing and simply label it. Then bring that attention and awareness back to the breath. Meditation is simply mindful breathing. Notice the breath, which carries the life-force energy through your entire being, but regard the space between the breaths. Watch the thoughts go by like clouds.

My greatest influence in the importance and ease of a meditation practice was my friend and dedicated spinning student at the time, actress Helen Hunt. She had a very rigorous work schedule between her television series and film career. Helen was intent on meditating twice daily for twenty minutes. The busier she was, the greater the importance to carve out the time. We would often spend twenty silent minutes together between scenes on the *Mad About You* set in meditation. In fact, Helen meditated in the limousine on the way to winning her Best Actress Oscar for her role in the movie *As Good as it Gets*. A true testament to the idea of detachment that comes from meditation. Meditation teaches us that our best day and our worst day are no different. She just so happened to win that day. The next day, she came to take my class and someone stole her spot. And so it goes. To further keep ourselves on track, we used the buddy system and started a weekly women's meditation group, and included other women. It's a great way to make practice consistent and spend time connecting with friends. Since that time, I have engaged with meditation myself in different ways. I've tried everything from a 4:00 AM Taoist visualization and standing meditation, to mantras and mala beads, meditation sangas, and kirtan. They have all worked, so it is not a matter of doing any one method correctly. The point is to keep a practice going and to make that space and time for yourself daily. Try a few, and see what resonates the most.

It doesn't have to be complicated. To start all you need is five minutes a day and a timer. Even if you only did five minutes daily, with one day off, you would have thirty meditation minutes under you belt at the end of just one week. Keep that up and by the end of the year you'll have twenty-four hours in silence for God to get a foot in the door. That is quite substantial. With so many meditation options to choose from, just choose one: mindful breathing, mantra, visualization, guided meditation. Try until you find what works for you. Don't be afraid to mix it up, like rotating crops that grow better when rotated every several months. Try one of the listed options today, and sample a new technique each day for the remainder of the 28-Day Revolution. (You only have four days to go!)

## ✺ ACTION CHECKLIST

### INTENTION: *Be.*

Today, as you move through the world, allow that to be sufficient. It is your birthright to take up space and to be present. There is nothing in particular you need to accomplish, no game face you have to put on, and no role you must play. You are enough as is.

### PLAYLIST: *Meditation Music*

The following is an album called Prana, by Craig Kohland & Shaman's Dream. The last track, "Storm of Prayers," is my favorite for Savasana. I mentioned this earlier in the book, so if you haven't checked it out yet, today's the day. It lasts eleven minutes and feels like heaven. You can use this entire album for your practice and finish in meditation. When the music ends, just sit in the sounds of silence.

"Prana"

"Honey In the Heart"

"Warming the Soul"

"Sacred Alchemy"

"Offerings"

"Holy Water"

"Storm of Prayers"

### YOGALOSOPHY ROUTINE VARIATION

Begin the routine with a five-minute meditation; end with a five-minute meditation. Simple.

### CARDIO OPTION

Instead of cardio today, meditate with a friend for twenty minutes. Set the tone for your meditation by turning the lights low and lighting a candle. If you have specific meditation music that works for you, you can turn that on as well. Or use today's playlist. Have a space that feels comfortable to both of you, and if you need pillows or blankets to soften your surroundings, feel free to make it as cozy as you like. Set a timer to go off after twenty minutes. If you would like to hold a crystal and share your thoughts for no more than five minutes at the end, you may. It is also nice to have hot tea for your postmeditation wrap-up. Sometimes our meditation group would make dinner together as well.

DAY 25

# MEDITATION EXERCISES

Try the following meditation exercises for five minutes each:

## MINDFUL BREATHING

Sit in Half-lotus (see Pose of the Day) or cross-legged with spine straight. Imagine a string extending through the top of your head, visualizing a line of energy through your spine. Unclench your jaw and touch the tongue to the roof of your mouth. Notice your natural breathing. As you notice the inhale at the nostrils, think "one" then exhale "one." Continue this through "ten" and begin again. It is normal for the thoughts to stray. When you notice, simply bring your attention back to the breathing. The mind is like a muscle; with practice, you will be able to hold your attention longer. Take five to twenty minutes here.

## VISUALIZATION

There are many different types of visualizations you can do, anything from imagining yourself in a peaceful garden to being near a body of water. Visualize your own scenario or try one of the following:

- Imagine your inner child emerging, and sit with that child. Hold her and tell her how much you love her, and that you will come back and visit. Then visualize angels holding your inner child for you. Enjoy this interaction and love.

- Imagine what it would feel like if you were completely loved and accepted exactly as you are, and just sit in that good feeling. Since it changes your brain chemistry when you smile, simply smile to yourself.

- Visualize pink bubbles around your thoughts and just let the pink bubbles float away. Or pop them!

## MANTRA

This is a word, or a string of words, that you can repeat to focus your mind and your thoughts in meditation. If you have mala beads, you can run your finger over each one and say the mantra. Mala has 108 beads on it, so do five rounds, repeating the mantra. "Om" is a simple word you can repeat. It need not be complicated.

# POSE OF THE DAY

## Half Lotus or Seated Meditation

Lotus (page 155) is a classic meditation pose in yoga, but not everyone can contort into Lotus. Try Half-lotus (below), or feel free to sit cross-legged and elevated on a meditation cushion. You may also sit on a chair, with both soles of the feet on the floor. When in meditation, sit with your spine straight. Your shoulders should be over your hips. Relax your face. Position your chin slightly down. You may touch the tongue to the roof of the mouth. Release yourself from any rigid expectation and just breathe.

### HALF LOTUS

Sit with legs extended, then hug the right knee into the chest and place the top of the right foot into the crease of the left leg so that your sole is facing the sky. Then cross your left ankle under your right knee. Make sure to do this for equal time on each side.

PHYSICAL BENEFITS: Stretches spine, ankles, and knee joints.

HEALING BENEFITS: Aids with sciatica and menstrual cramps. Stimulates the function of the pelvis, spine, and bladder.

EMOTIONAL ASPECTS: Helps to calm the mind and enliven a meditative state.

MODIFICATIONS: If your knees or ankles are bothered, simply sit cross-legged.

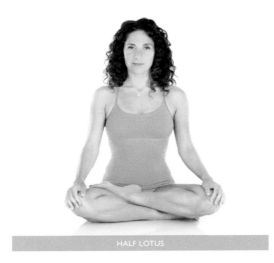

HALF LOTUS

## EXTRA CREDIT: *Tips for meditation.*

Start a meditation group, find a meditation group or kirtan, or look into a vipassana retreat. Tips for meditation:

- Create a ritual around meditation: Light a candle.

- Play a song like "Storm of Prayers" by Craig Kohland & Shaman's Dream.

- Count mala beads while you repeat a mantra.

- Keep your spine straight.

- Use the breath as a point of focus to bring your thoughts back to the present.

- When thoughts come, watch them go by like clouds.

- Set a time to be mindful and observe yourself daily.

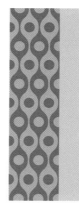

■ **JOURNAL**
Write a poem.

■ **GRATITUDE LIST**

■ **BREATHING EXERCISE**
For the next four days, replace your breathing exercise with meditation.

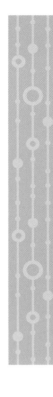

# Recipe: TONYA'S CHAI TEA

I will never forget my dear friend Tonya Crowe, who made me chai tea for the first time in the early '90s. I have been a convert ever since. I use almond milk instead of dairy. The treat of the day is that you get to have black tea. Enjoy!

**1 cup almond milk**
**1 black tea bag**
**3 pods cardamom**
**1 piece cinnamon bark**
**2 cloves**
**honey, to taste**

In a pot, bring almond milk, cardamom, cinnamon, cloves, and honey to a boil, and add tea bag.

Steep and drink this delicious treat. Since this has caffeine, you can either use a decaf option or make sure to drink it in the morning!

# DAY 26

## BECOME A BLISS ARTIST
### *Your Body is Your Art*

We are all artists; everything we ingest and do or feel and think creates our physical body—our own work of art. You have been re-creating this body, reshaping and resculpting it mentally, emotionally, and physically. Sometimes the more we think on something, the more confused we become. A calm and focused mind is not always reached through sitting in meditation or physical activity; sometimes we have to approach things from a different angle. Not head-on, but through the back door; through right-brained creativity.

Immersion in art is a meditation, an expression of something words cannot capture. You don't have to be Picasso or Monet to put paint to canvas and express your artistic soul.

Have you ever noticed that every child is an inspired artist? I remember reading in Henry Miller's art book that each child paints perfectly composed pictures. It's when judgment and a discerning eye enter a room that we become inhibited and distort our natural expression in order to fit a mold. My own mother was a great artist, and one of the first things she taught me, other than strokes and shading, was a good habit that I have been trying to break ever since. My mother taught me to color inside the lines, just like she did.

> *"All children are artists. The problem is how to remain an artist when [s]he grows up."*
> — PABLO PICASSO

I was touted as a great artist among teachers and friends. My shading and strokes were enviable, my perspective and rendering incredibly lifelike, yet I hadn't even accessed my spirit's true nature. As I grew up, I found that my true style is much more childlike and that is how I enjoy painting today. I had an art teacher tell me in school once that there are no mistakes, only happy accidents.

Art is therapeutic, and it is another wordless way to let our thoughts and mind go, while we allow our emotional wisdom to flow. I call this being a bliss artist. Joy is a side effect of giving yourself a place to experience the full range of your human emotions. You may wonder what painting can do for your Y28 Revolution. Will this actually help you have a better body?

Living a holistic life of health and wellness requires all facets of yourself. After all, at this point, sugar is probably no longer your ideal go-to pal for self-soothing the emotions that ebb and flow through you and fuel your life. The key to finding true joy and happiness is not to deny yourself what you feel, but to transform and transmute that depth through your creativity. When used as a vehicle, art that is inspired by your emotional wisdom brings you closer to spirit.

Sometimes, picking up a blank canvas and expressing yourself wordlessly is means for meditation. You are already a bliss artist, and your body is your art, as you have been re-creating it over the last twenty-six days. It is as if you have been a sculptor, sanding away with your sandpaper and chiseling with your tools to reveal the true form that was waiting to be revealed all of this time. So you are the sculptor, the alchemist, the mystic, the artist. Take a moment to delight in your creation, whatever the phase. I hope you have colored outside of the lines!

## ✿ ACTION CHECKLIST

**INTENTION:** *Channel your bliss.*

Whatever you are feeling is okay because you can use it for your art! (See Extra Credit.)

**PLAYLIST:** *Silence*

No music today. See if you can tolerate the silence and enjoy no music during your meditation or yoga today. Some of my best practices have been in the presence of natural surround-sound.

**YOGALOSOPHY ROUTINE VARIATION**

Follow the routine as always, but add meditation to the routine.

**CARDIO OPTION**

Walking meditation. Walking on the treadmill still works. Remember that you are a sculptor and that you are sanding your body down to reveal the beautiful shape and work of art that you are.

DAY 26

# POSE OF THE DAY

## HAPPY BABY

Lie on your back and hug your knees to your chest. Hold on to the outsides of your feet. Open your knees to the outside of your side body, bringing the knees up toward the armpits. Flex your feet to aim the soles of the feet up to the ceiling, aligning your ankles and knees so that your shins are perpendicular to the floor. Release your tailbone toward the floor, almost arching your back. Slightly tuck your chin so that your spine is nice and elongated. Hold for six to ten breaths.

**PHYSICAL BENEFITS:** Stretches hips and groin.

**HEALING BENEFITS:** Relieves stress and fatigue.

**EMOTIONAL ASPECTS:** Opens hips, which, as you know, are programmed to receive.

**MODIFICATIONS:** Try using a folded blanket under your head if your chin is jutting upward. May use straps to wrap around your feet if you cannot reach the feet comfortably.

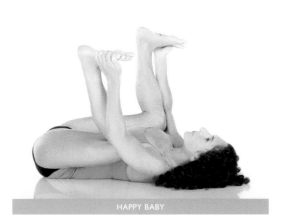
HAPPY BABY

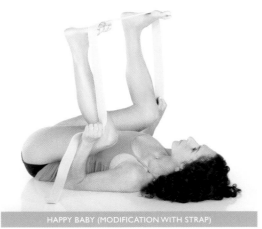
HAPPY BABY (MODIFICATION WITH STRAP)

## EXTRA CREDIT: *Express yourself through art!*

Find a visual art form you can enjoy—painting, drawing, coloring—and delight in it for at least ten minutes. You don't have to show anybody what you create. It's just for you.

- **JOURNAL**
  No journal today. The painting is a replacement for your journaling.

- **GRATITUDE LIST**

- **MEDITATION**
  Choose from any of the options from Day 25, or sit for ten minutes before and after your routine. Remember: Sitting in meditation is a muscle of the mind. You will get stronger with consistent practice. It will get easier and you will see results just like with physical exercise. This will replace the breathing exercises for the remainder of the program.

# Recipe: PAINTED FRUIT

Food is art! That's right, paint your food green and get messy! I got this recipe from one of my closest friends who has embraced and truly lives a lifestyle of joy. Laura Harrelson, wife of main yogi Woody Harrelson, is one of my besties. And she feeds me very well. This dessert or breakfast dish will knock your socks off. It is a masterpiece.

1 heaping tablespoon raw almond butter
1 heaping tablespoon raw tahini
1 teaspoon agave nectar
1 tablespoon fresh-squeezed lemon juice
1 tablespoon hempseed oil
3 tablespoons spirulina powder
½ teaspoon ground cinnamon
¼ teaspoon Celtic sea salt
½ cup coconut water

In a small bowl, mix almond butter, tahini, agave, lemon juice, cinnamon, and hempseed oil together until creamy. Slowly stir in spirulina powder. If mix starts to get too thick, start stirring in the juice and then add the remaining spirulina. Mix to desired consistency. You may forego the juice, depending on desired thickness.

Pour or spoon the mix over freshly cut fruit (banana, mango, papaya, heaps of berries). Garnish with more cinnamon and dried coconut shavings. The paint doesn't last very long, so consume immediately, share with friends, or store in the fridge! May be served with chopped almonds for added crunch.

# DAY 27

## FIND YOUR INNER RHYTHM

### *Life Is a Dance*

**Y**esterday you found your creative skills by painting a picture. Today you can channel the physical creativity through the art of music and dance, and use that as your meditation, yoga, and cardio routine.

Think about your favorite song. Often, great art or music that we connect with was inspired by love or born out of deep grief or sadness. Heartbreak produces some of our greatest poetry and the most popular songs that bond us together. I have always been attracted to music, yet I have not developed any skills with instruments or through my voice, so my way of musical expression has been to move my body and use it as the instrument. I often feel like the music is accessing me so that it can vibrate through me. Music, like art, is subjective. Just as a child always paints a perfect picture, so does she always move in the most organic and expressive ways.

> *"Dance is the hidden language of the soul of the body."*
> — MARTHA GRAHAM

Today is all about the music in you. Would you like to bang on a tabletop? Dance wildly to music that moves you? Do you want to make a playlist that represents the soundtrack to your current life? Or would you just like to have a day to let your "inner" music play?

As we begin to come to the end of our Y28 Revolution, we let the rules go and start to live our revolution. I ask you today to be the dancer. Express your art as you feel it in your body. There are no rules for your day today. You should sleep when you feel like it, eat when you need to, and go with the flow. You know now that your body's natural state is health, and your job is to start listening, allowing your body to fall into place naturally. Be easy on yourself while you are continuing with your routine. Release yourself from rigidity. Whatever happens today, it is exactly as it should be. Nature and the universe are conspiring to help you. Go with it.

## ✺ ACTION CHECKLIST

**INTENTION:** *Follow the rhythm.*

Everything has a rhythm and a right way. Breath is your body's internal rhythm section. Allow the rhythm of the day unfold to you. Whatever comes is just the way it should be. Trust that.

**PLAYLIST:** *Personal Mix*

Make your own playlist today. Find the songs that have some of your favorite lyrics. Find the music and words that speak to you.

**YOGALOSOPHY ROUTINE VARIATION**

Have a great film on when you practice, or listen to an audio track of poetry by one of your favorite poets. Be creative and messy today.

**CARDIO OPTION**

It's a "dancing around in your living room" kind of day. Can you do it for forty minutes?

DAY 27

# POSE OF THE DAY

## COBBLER'S POSE

Put the soles of your feet together. Let your knees drop open; release the sides of your waist. Open your hips. As you release the hips, the lower back and spine will lengthen. Take a deep inhale and on the exhale, fold forward. You can support yourself if you need to with a pillow underneath each knee. You can stay seated with the hands behind you to lengthen the lower back. If you have flexibility in your hips, you may be able to fold all the way forward.

PHYSICAL BENEFITS: Eases back pain, and uterine and urinary tract conditions. Stretches inner thighs, knees, and groin.

HEALING BENEFITS: Stimulates bladder, kidneys, ovaries, and circulation.

EMOTIONAL ASPECTS: Releases tension and fear that we hold in the hips.

MODIFICATIONS: May place pillows under each knee for support.

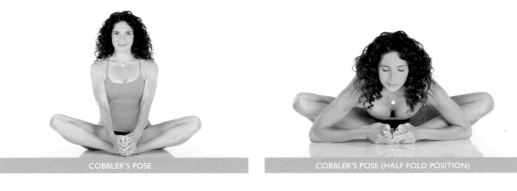

COBBLER'S POSE

COBBLER'S POSE (HALF FOLD POSITION)

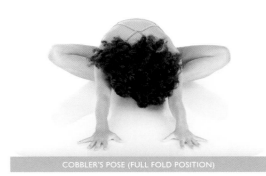

COBBLER'S POSE (FULL FOLD POSITION)

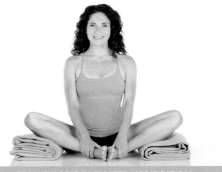

COBBLER'S POSE (SUPPORTED MODIFICATION)

## EXTRA CREDIT: *Break the rules.*

Have a glass of wine at the end of your practice today or put your feet up. Maybe you want to have the TV on during your practice. No rules. Behave like the artist in you would.

### ■ JOURNAL

Write a poem or a song to your body (or from your body to you). Yes. It's a fun exercise. Remember: You alone are writing and reading this. Put it in an envelope and date it as DO NOT OPEN until some later time. Seal it, and do not open until the end date. I cannot tell you how many beautiful love poems and letters I have planted for myself over the years.

### ■ GRATITUDE LIST

How do I love myself? Let me count the five ways.

### ■ MEDITATION

## *Recipe:* WHITEFISH IN BEAUJOLAIS SAUCE

This recipe has alcohol in it (but it gets burned off during the cooking process). However, feel free to have a glass of wine with dinner (see Extra Credit). Relax a little!

3 pounds whitefish
1 finely chopped onion
1 tablespoon parsley
2 cloves garlic
5 tablespoons olive oil
1 tablespoon unbleached flour
1½ cups water
2 glasses red wine
Salt
Bay leaf

Cut fish into 1-inch pieces, sprinkle with salt. Put on a large plate. Saute chopped onion and garlic in olive oil in a heavy saucepan. Sprinkle the flour over the oil as you stir. Add 1½ cups water and 2 glasses of wine. Add parsley and bay leaf. Simmer for 15 minutes. Add pieces of fish. Cover and cook for 15 minutes more.

# DAY 28

## RELEASE

### *Retreat, Release, and Let Go*

**Y**ou made it! How exciting! You persevered to Day 28. Doesn't it feel excellent? Following a program like this for the past twenty-eight days allows you to experience what it is to feel a sense of completion, which is my absolute favorite feeling. I have always loved the grand finale, taking my final bow, even finishing off a bottle of shampoo. There is always a sense of accomplishment when you achieve your goal, yet there is also a sense of loss as we release all that we have worked for and say good-bye to our daily activities. You have fulfilled your commitment.

> *"Tweet Tweet Tweet. Free Free Free."*
> — LLOYD INGBER

After everything, after all of the work and the meditating and the playing, just releasing and letting go can be the most challenging of all actions. Perhaps this is new behavior. Enjoy this. Be as present as you can. Honor the road you have traveled and all that you have explored in yourself. You know your mind, body, heart, and spirit so much better now. You have met with your darkness, as well as with the go-getter and the artist within you. You have danced with your little child and you have been diligent with your commitment. You have tricked, cajoled, encouraged, felt your way through, struggled, pretended, and visualized. You have cheated and honored and skipped over, and somehow you are right here, with nothing in particular to do, except say good-bye for now and release.

When we begin a yoga practice, we often begin in Child's Pose, setting an intention for ourselves and making a decision about how we will view our experience of the practice. As you begin in Child's Pose, you then contort and move your body through multiple postures, in some ways mimicking the process of life. That is why the final pose is a resting pose: Savasana, or Corpse Pose. You may forget that your body does its best work when you are sleeping. When you're "doing nothing," you are actually allowing your body to integrate all the work you have completed. That's why in yoga, Savasana is considered the most important of all the poses. In the end, you are not your body. Your body processes and is a container and a vehicle for the lessons you have learned; yet in the end, we practice what we will ultimately do at the finish line, and let go of the body.

It was not easy to watch my father struggle through his cancer. He had always been so diligent about his routine and his consistent self-care and exploration of his body. One of the most difficult moments that I experienced was watching my father, who had once been so in control of his body, experience an allergic reaction to some medication while getting chemotherapy. I remember he could not speak through his shivering. He looked at me with fear in his eyes, as if to say, "What the hell?" I imagined how out of control he felt, considering he had self-diagnosed his own cancer by tuning in during his yogic practices. I simply looked at him and called upon my teaching skills. All I could do was to contain his experience by witnessing and stating the obvious. "Just another way to explore being in the body." I looked him straight in the eye and rubbed his feet to create some friction and some heat.

It was hard for my family to accept that this Ingber superpower was dying. I had called hospice a month before, and they talked me through the final part of the process, which is that the respiratory system starts to shut down and the person seems to have a cold. When I called my dad's house to check on him, and my twelve-year-old half sister said, "Poppa has a cold," I knew I had to get over to his house to say good-bye to him. When I got there, he seemed out of it and he mentioned that there was a "man on his shoulder." I remembered a story my father had told me about his own father's death. He told me he knew his father was dying because he saw the Angel of Death come into the room. I did not see anything, but I knew whom my father was talking about.

My father, who was drugged up on medication, said, and repeated twice: "Tweet tweet tweet, free free free." That was at 5:30 PM on a Saturday night. A mere seven hours later, we were all at the hospital, with his prophecy coming true. His wife and my brother Dave were on either side of him. At last, everyone was ready to let go, and I was finally free to say good-bye to my dad for good. It was 1:00 AM. I will say that watching the dying process is similar to the birthing process. I have only been witness to one birth, but this was a reminder that death is another gateway.

How do we let go? In the end, we are not in control, so how can we be present to the unraveling when, for our whole lives, we have felt in control and somehow in charge of these bodies. I watched as my father struggled, drugged up, half-conscious, speaking partially coherently and half in brain babble. He requested to sit up, regardless of the tumors that were strangling him at both ends. I have actually heard that yogic masters like to die sitting up, with a straight spine, so that they may leave through the crown of the head. I know that my father had been a practitioner of some pretty esoteric Taoist yoga. The three of us hauled him to a chair. We pushed and pulled: "One, two, three!" and got him up. He sat, but could not stay, so we had to move him back to the table, and he lay down. "One, two, three, pshhhh." He tried to push himself out of his body; maybe his spirit would be able to be shot out of his physical body? Not happening. Then I thought he was trying to get up and walk out of his body.

"Dad, are you dying?"

"Yes."

"Well you can't take your body with you."

My gosh, it was so difficult for me to watch his process as I was trying to tell him how to die!

He said, "It's a process of opening up." Ultimately he was just a human being, and once they gave him a morphine drip, he was able to detach enough from his body to stop trying to control it any more, and he let go.

My father passed at 7:17 AM while I was out of the room. Just the way it was supposed to happen. I was on the phone, letting a coworker know that I was going to have to cancel my 7:30 AM spinning class. When I walked into the room on the most beautiful August Sunday morning I could remember in Los Angeles, I looked at his body. I scanned it from top to bottom, from his hair transplant scars and the tattoos that covered it, to the wisdom teeth he had removed; all the way down to his beautiful feet and his one fungal toenail. This man who had been carried by this body, who loved and had a relationship with his body . . . and in the end, here it was—a mere suitcase. I felt all of his energy actually spread out evenly at the top of the hospital room. In the end, we all must leave the body behind. Live this day like it was your last. Tweet Tweet Tweet. Free Free Free.

In a way, my entire life as a yoga instructor, fitness advisor, and wellness expert was born from my father's example, both positive and negative. I will never forget that this man left me with far more than I ever knew that he gave. I bear witness, I receive, I embody, I honor, pass along, and release. This journey in the body is so brief. The time when you are able to have the willpower to stick with something and the strength to be able to follow through and carry it out is a small window, indeed. Use your energy wisely, and be full in your expression. Appreciate every moment. I am sure that in the end, it will all be exactly as it should be. Integrate every facet of yourself by loving and honoring through this most amazing gift: The vehicle of your human body.

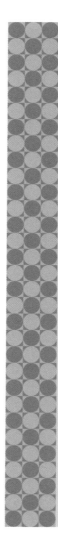

## ✧ ACTION CHECKLIST

**INTENTION:** *Release and let go.*

Live this day as if it were your last.

**PLAYLIST:** *Release*

I made this playlist, in part for my dad. You get the idea.

"Let Go," Frou Frou

"Ends," Everlast

"Release Me," Pearl Jam

"I Still Haven't Found What I'm Looking For," U2

"Baba Hanuman," Krishna Das

"Om Namah Shivaya," Wah!

**YOGALOSOPHY ROUTINE VARIATION**

Do the thirty-minute routine for the last time. Include the seven-minute stretch at the end. See Stretch Series (page 236).

**CARDIO OPTION**

Victory lap. A short walk. Whatever you need to feel complete. Twenty minutes of cardio will do.

DAY 28

# POSE OF THE DAY

## SAVASANA/CORPSE POSE

This is the final resting pose in yoga. It is the most important pose of the day because it is where the body integrates all of the hard work it did—all of the balance, strength, and stretching. This pose allows your body to process all of this information at the end of the routine.

Lie on your back. Allow the feet to flop open to the sides or prop your knees with a rolled up towel or bolster. Press the shoulders down and spin the palms upwards so that the chest and shoulders are open. Allow your body to feel heavy, as if it will make an impression in the floor when you get up. Allow your jaw to go slack and your face to relax. Breathe naturally. Stay here for five to thirty minutes today. Try not to fall asleep, but to drift in a subtle awareness. When you are ready to come out of this, begin to lengthen your breath and start to move your fingers and toes. Roll over to your right side and curl into a ball. When you are ready, press yourself up to a seated, cross-legged position and bring your palms together in prayer position at your heart.

At the end of a yoga practice, the teacher will say "namaste," which means: The divine within me salutes the divine that is within you.

NAMASTE.

**PHYSICAL BENEFITS:** Allows the body to integrate and reset itself after any practice.

**HEALING BENEFITS:** Lowers blood pressure, heart rate. Decreases muscle tension. Improves focus.

**EMOTIONAL ASPECTS:** Enhances self-confidence. Allows detachment and observation. Aids awareness in release and letting go. Brightens mood.

**MODIFICATIONS:** If uncomfortable for your lower back, try placing a pillow or a rolled up towel underneath the backs of the knees.

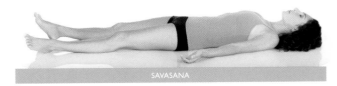
SAVASANA

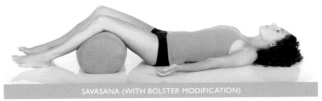
SAVASANA (WITH BOLSTER MODIFICATION)

# EXTRA CREDIT: *Let go.*

After your routine, do a fifteen-minute Savasana (or longer, if you like).

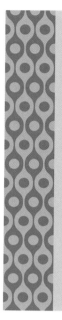

- **JOURNAL**

Congratulate yourself. You did it. Write a thank you note to your body, for all that it does for you.

- **GRATITUDE LIST**

Be grateful that you can breathe, that your limbs move; for the beautiful sky, life's experiences and how you keep on trying, the people in your life who relate with you for better or worse, and the mystery that threads us all together; if you have your sight, your sight—if you don't, then your sense of touch—when you wake up, be grateful the birds are singing and the sun is shining. Or it's raining and wet and beautiful. Life is good.

- **MEDITATION**

Remain in Savasana/Corpse Pose as long as you want.

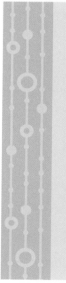

## *Recipe:* MY ALMOND SHAKE RECIPE

Eat minimally today. You are not your body. Eat smaller meals. Only what you need. Here's a delicious liquid meal:

**Almond milk (about 12 oz., but add or reduce according to your preference)**
**2 tablespoons almond butter (or to taste)**
**Cinnamon**
**Ice**
**½ packet Stevia**
**½ frozen banana**

Blend with ice to desired consistency and enjoy the delicious concoction.

PART 3

# Resources

# YOGALOSOPHY ROUTINE EXTRAS

The basic Yogalosophy Routine is the foundation of your workout every day. However, some days call for variations in the routine. The "Fully Loaded" workout below is a variation that builds on the basic routine, incorporating additional strength and balance exercises. This 55-minute routine is a well-rounded workout that opens with Sun Salutations and closes with Stretches, bringing you full circle through poses and toners that work both your body *and* your mind.

## THE "FULLY LOADED" WORKOUT

Combine the following series of poses and toners in one complete workout. You'll find full instructions for the extra exercises on the following pages. For the Yogalosophy Routine poses and toners, please see pages 9 through 24.

- Sun Salutation

- Strength Series

- Balance Challenge

- Yogalosophy Routine

- Stretch Series

## Sun Salutation

### MOUNTAIN POSE

Begin with feet together and palms together in front of your heart. Close your eyes. Get centered. As you inhale, sweep the arms over your head and prepare for Forward Bend.

### FORWARD BEND

As you exhale, hinge at the hips and fold forward. Again, inhale, keep the palms on the floor, or bring you hands up to the knees; raise your chest halfway forward, flatten your spine. Move to Plank.

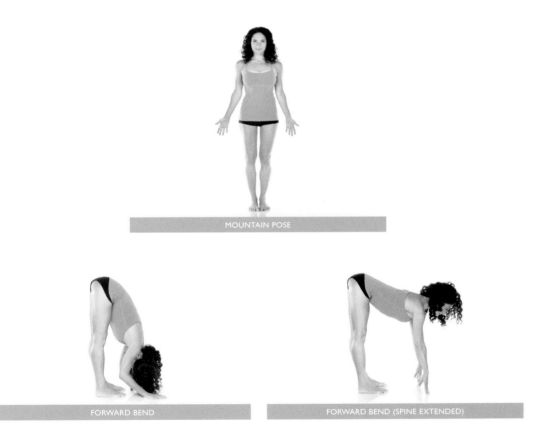

MOUNTAIN POSE

FORWARD BEND

FORWARD BEND (SPINE EXTENDED)

### PLANK

Exhale, step back to Plank, holding your body straight, as if you're at the top of a push-up. Look straight ahead. Inhale. Exhale, lower down, hugging the elbows in close to your body, making sure your belly, chest, and chin lower at the same time.

### UPWARD FACING DOG

Inhale, lift the heart up (shoulders roll back away from the ears) into Cobra or Upward Facing Dog.

### DOWNWARD FACING DOG

Exhale, press back to Downward Facing Dog. Take five breaths. At the end of the last exhale, look up to the hands. Step the feet to the hands. Prepare to return to Mountain Pose. Inhale, look up, bringing your torso halfway up, chest forward, spine flat. Exhale, fold down. Inhale, press the feet into the mat and firm your thighs to rise up with a flat back to Mountain Pose. Exhale, press the palms together at the heart. Repeat five times.

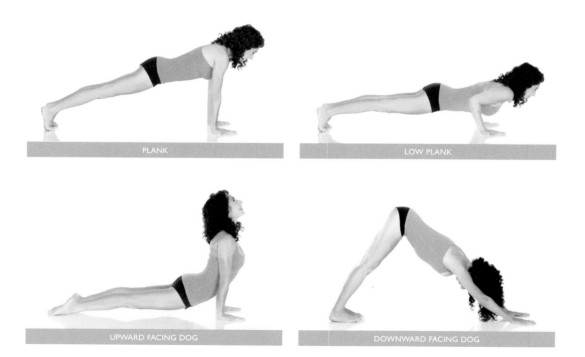

PLANK

LOW PLANK

UPWARD FACING DOG

DOWNWARD FACING DOG

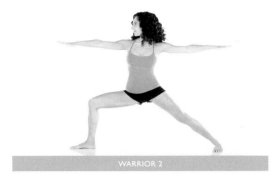

WARRIOR 2

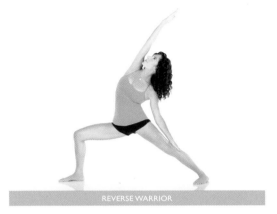

REVERSE WARRIOR

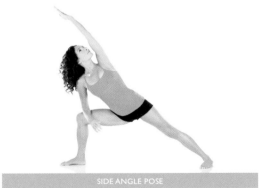

SIDE ANGLE POSE

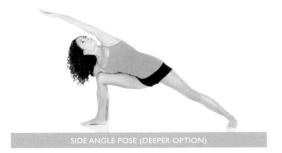

SIDE ANGLE POSE (DEEPER OPTION)

## Strength Series

### WARRIOR 2

Step your feet about three to five feet apart. Turn your right toes out to the right, and line your right heel with your back (left) arch. Bend your right (front) knee to a ninety-degree angle. Extend your arms out to shoulder level and gaze down the center of your hand. Your shoulders, hips, and knees should be in aligned. Take five to ten deep breaths. Move to Reverse Warrior.

### REVERSE WARRIOR

Slide your left (back) hand down the left hamstring as you extend your right arm up and over, aligning your biceps with your cheek as you gaze upward and reach back. Five to ten deep breaths. Return to Warrior 2.

### SIDE ANGLE POSE

Bring your front (right) forearm onto your right thigh. Pressing away from the thigh will create more space and elongate your neck. Extend your left arm up and over. Take five to ten breaths. Return to Warrior 2 and repeat on the left side.

# Balance Challenge

## MOUNTAIN POSE

Stand with your feet together and palms in prayer position, ground your feet by spreading the toes. Feel the floor supporting you. Distribute the weight evenly; do not allow the arches of your feet to cave in. Firm your thighs to lift your kneecaps. Drop your tailbone down toward your heels. Lift up out of your waist. Roll your shoulders up, back, around and down, as you glide the shoulder blades down by the spine. Root down through your legs, like the roots of a tree. Extend long, out through the top of your head for ten breaths.

## KNEE TO CHEST

From Mountain Pose, lift your right leg and clasp your hands just below the knee. Maintain your balance as you draw your knee in to your chest, while keeping your spine straight.

## TREE POSE

From knee to chest, turn your right knee out as you draw the sole of your right foot to the inner thigh or calf of your left standing leg. Press the sole of your foot and the inner thigh together. Steady your gaze and connect with your breathing. Keep your right knee turning out as you gently tuck your tailbone. With your palms in prayer position at your heart, press them together and extend them up and over your head. Extend a line of energy out through the crown of the head. Hold for five to ten breaths and repeat on side two.

## WARRIOR 3

Find a gazing point and fix your gaze. As you focus on your breath, begin to lean forward shifting your weight onto your left leg and lean forward until your leg and torso are on the same line, like the letter T. Make sure your standing leg is straight, then find extension out through the crown of your head and your back extended heel. Extend your arms out to the sides. Breathe.

## LEG LIFT

From Warrior 3, bring your hands to your hips and slowly begin to bring your body back into an upright position. Sweep the right leg all the way through and try not to let your right leg touch the floor. Extend it straight out in front of you as you stand upright. Draw the lower abdominals in.

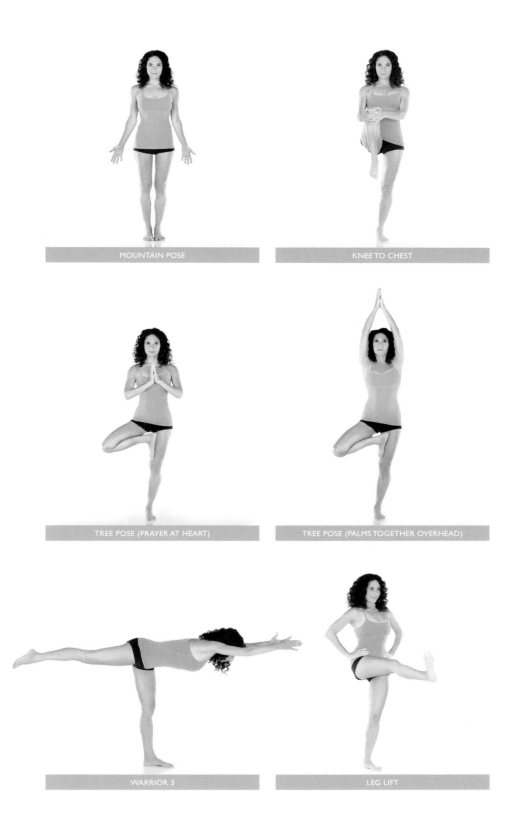

MOUNTAIN POSE

KNEE TO CHEST

TREE POSE (PRAYER AT HEART)

TREE POSE (PALMS TOGETHER OVERHEAD)

WARRIOR 3

LEG LIFT

## Stretch Series

### LOW LUNGE

From Downward Facing Dog, raise your left leg behind you. Flex your foot to extend out through your heel. Internally rotate your thigh. Both hip bones should be level and aiming toward the floor. Step your foot between your hands so that the toenails and fingernails are in alignment. Go ahead and drop your right knee to the floor. From here, sink your hips down, let your sacrum get really heavy. Feel the stretch in your front hip flexor. Breathe.

### PIGEON

From the Low Lunge, keep your hands on the floor and lift your left foot. Bend your left knee in front of you and slowly lower down, drawing the sole of your foot to the groin area or inner thigh of your right leg. The hips should be facing squarely to the floor. Your left knee is out slightly to the left of your left shoulder, and your foot is aiming toward your right shoulder. Fold forward and breathe.

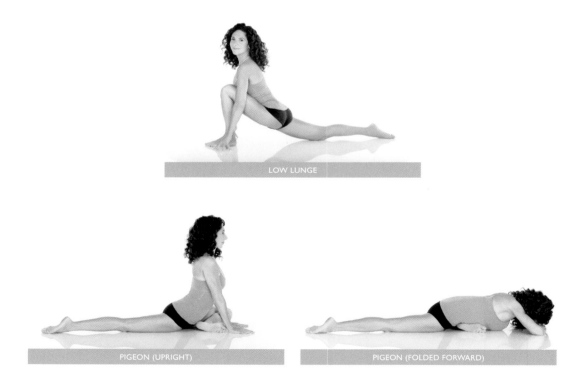

LOW LUNGE

PIGEON (UPRIGHT)

PIGEON (FOLDED FORWARD)

## SEATED FORWARD BEND

When you have completed Pigeon on the left side, walk your hands back, lean to the side of your bent leg, and sweep your back leg out in front. Extend both legs now. Shake out your legs in front of you and fold forward.

## SEATED ONE-LEGGED FORWARD BEND

Bring the sole of your right foot to the groin area or inner thigh of your left leg. Keep your left leg straight and extended long. Inhale, arms up, and extend your spine. Exhale, fold forward, and reach for the foot. If you can't reach, use a towel to wrap underneath your foot and use the leverage to draw your chest toward the top of your foot. Breathe. Five to ten breaths. Rise to sitting. Switch sides.

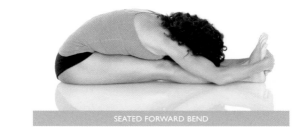
SEATED FORWARD BEND

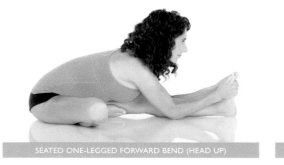
SEATED ONE-LEGGED FORWARD BEND (HEAD UP)

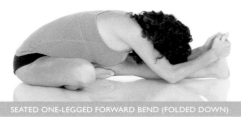
SEATED ONE-LEGGED FORWARD BEND (FOLDED DOWN)

## COBBLER'S POSE

Bring the soles of your feet together. Let your knees drop open, release the sides of your waist. Open your hips. As you release your hips, your lower back and spine will lengthen. Take a deep inhale and on the exhale, fold forward. You can support yourself if you need to with a pillow underneath each knee. You can stay seated with your hands behind you to lengthen the lower back. If you have flexibility in your hips you may be able to fold all the way forward.

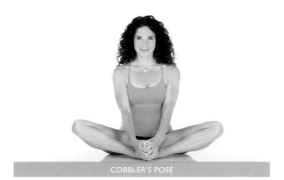

COBBLER'S POSE

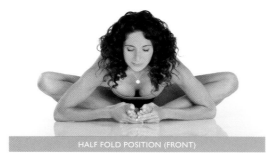

HALF FOLD POSITION (FRONT)

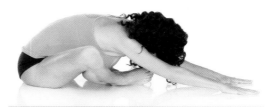

FULL FOLD POSITION (SIDE)

## SEATED FORWARD FOLD

With both legs extended, move the fleshy part of your tush away to the sides. Ground your sit bones to the floor. On the inhale, extend your arms up and reach for the sky, and on the exhale, reach your chest toward the tops of your feet and fold down. If you can reach your feet, use the leverage to draw your body down. If not, use a band or belt to increase the stretch. Breathe here. Rise back up to sitting.

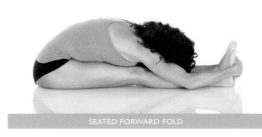

SEATED FORWARD FOLD

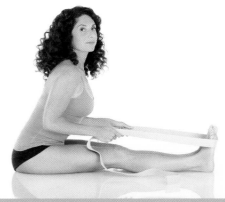

SEATED FORWARD FOLD (MODIFICATION WITH STRAP)

# DIET PLANS

The mind-body transformation that comes from participating in the Y28 Revolution requires a holistic approach to health and wellness, so the food you choose to eat plays a major role in achieving your goals. The three options outlined in this section accommodate just about all diet preferences and requirements, from gluten-free and vegetarian, to low-carb omnivore. There really is something for everyone! But as I mentioned in the beginning of the book, it's important to stick to one option in order to maximize the benefits of the program.

For each diet plan, I have included a grocery list of foods that you will need to have on hand in your pantry and refrigerator. Your initial shop will probably be the most expensive until you get your kitchen stocked with all the proper oils, condiments, etc. Once you get into a groove, you will mostly be buying produce, which is actually less expensive than the processed foods you may have been buying in the past. But you get more bang and nutrition for your buck! You won't need to eat as much, and you will be ingesting LIVE, FRESH, food, versus dead, processed food.

To keep your food as fresh as possible, shop for three to four days' worth of food at a time. Most of the recipes in these meal plans make between two to four servings, so make sure you take that into account. Since some of the meals use leftovers from dinner for lunch, it will not go to waste. Batch-cooking food is a great way to ensure you have plenty of delicious healthy food on hand so that you are not left starving or tempted to make a choice that is not good for you. Make sure to always buy organic, especially with dairy or animal products. It's best to get organic vegetables too, but for produce with a thick skin, like avocados, it's not always necessary.

Most of the recipes in these plans are simple to make, but don't be afraid to use your own recipes! It's important to eat as many of the foods on the "foods allowed" grocery list as you can, so go ahead and get creative with your cooking. Also, don't be afraid to interchange any of these meals as you see fit. Have breakfast for dinner and vice-versa! The Japanese traditionally have soup for breakfast, as it's an awesome and alkalizing way to start the day, so step out of your breakfast box and try something new!

## DIET PLAN A: *Clean*

To help develop the meal plan for this program, I turned to Vikki Krinsky, an L.A.-based private chef with a background in nutrition who caters to the culinary needs of celebrities, athletes, and other health-minded professionals. I like Vikki's approach because it's all about balance. Her theory is that a portion-based meal plan that limits certain foods but doesn't completely eliminate them allows each individual to maintain a healthy lifestyle while managing their cravings. Her reasoning makes sense. She explains, "We are programmed to want what we can't have, which is why I'm a great believer in moderation." Amen to that! I know firsthand that this food program will energize and empower you throughout the day to achieve your goals while controlling your urges. What's not to like about that?

# PLAN A: *Clean* GROCERY LIST

This is the general shopping list of all the foods you can eat on the Clean plan. Buying certain foods in bulk, such as nuts and grains, will save you money. Remember to buy organic and stay away from packaged, processed foods whenever possible.

## PROTEINS:
- [ ] Almond Milk
- [ ] Beef (fillets)
- [ ] Chicken (skinless breasts)
- [ ] Eggs/egg whites
- [ ] Salmon
- [ ] Shrimp (cooked)
- [ ] Tempeh
- [ ] Tilapia
- [ ] Tuna (canned, water-packed)
- [ ] Turkey (deli slices, sodium-free)
- [ ] Turkey (ground white meat)
- [ ] Veggie burgers

## DAIRY:
- [ ] Cheddar cheese (white)
- [ ] Cottage cheese (low fat)
- [ ] Goat cheese
- [ ] Greek yogurt (nonfat)
- [ ] Swiss cheese (lite)

## NUTS & SEEDS
(RAW ONLY):
- [ ] Almonds, cashews, hazelnuts, macadamias, pecans, pine nuts, walnuts
- [ ] Chia seeds, flax seeds, hemp seeds, pumpkin seeds, sesame seeds, sunflower seeds

- [ ] Raw nut and seed butters (no sugar added): almond, cashew, macadamia, pumpkin, sunflower, tahini

## GRAINS:
- [ ] Brown rice
- [ ] Bulgur
- [ ] Gluten-free brown rice tortillas
- [ ] Gluten-free China black rice bread
- [ ] Gluten-free crackers/ rice crackers
- [ ] Oatmeal
- [ ] Protein pretzels
- [ ] Quinoa
- [ ] Rice cakes
- [ ] Wheatberries

## OILS:
- [ ] Coconut oil
- [ ] Earth Balance "butter" (made with olive oil)
- [ ] Olive oil (extra-virgin)
- [ ] Olive oil spray
- [ ] Sesame oil (toasted and plain)

## VEGETABLES:
- [ ] Arugula
- [ ] Asparagus
- [ ] Avocado
- [ ] Bell peppers (red and green)

- [ ] Broccoli/broccolini
- [ ] Butter lettuce
- [ ] Carrots/baby carrots
- [ ] Cauliflower
- [ ] Celery
- [ ] Cucumber
- [ ] Edamame
- [ ] Garlic
- [ ] Jalapeno
- [ ] Kale
- [ ] Leeks
- [ ] Mushrooms
- [ ] Olives
- [ ] Onions (red, yellow, scallions)
- [ ] Pickles (baby dill)
- [ ] Shallots
- [ ] Shredded lettuce
- [ ] Spinach
- [ ] Sweet potato
- [ ] Tomatoes (regular, roma, cherry; canned and diced, sauce)
- [ ] Zucchini

## FRESH HERBS:
- [ ] Basil
- [ ] Chives
- [ ] Cilantro
- [ ] Dill
- [ ] Mint
- [ ] Parsley
- [ ] Tarragon

## LEGUMES:
- [ ] Beluga lentils
- [ ] Black beans
- [ ] Cannellini beans
- [ ] Chickpeas
- [ ] Kidney beans
- [ ] White beans

## FRUITS:
- [ ] Apples
- [ ] Bananas
- [ ] Blackberries
- [ ] Blueberries
- [ ] Lemons
- [ ] Oranges
- [ ] Pears
- [ ] Raspberries

## CONDIMENTS:
- [ ] Balsamic vinegar
- [ ] Dijon mustard
- [ ] Distilled vinegar
- [ ] Honey mustard
- [ ] Red wine vinegar

## MONDAY

*Breakfast:*

**GREEN-HERB OMELET
WITH GOAT CHEESE**

5 egg whites
½ cup fresh spinach
3 tablespoons diced green pepper
2 tablespoons freshly chopped dill
2 tablespoons chopped chives
2 tablespoons fresh goat cheese
1 piece toasted gluten-free bread

Place bread in toaster. Lightly spray pan, and heat on medium low. Add egg whites to cover pan. Once solid white, add all the ingredients on one side of omelet. Gently fold other side over and keep on heat for a minute longer to melt cheese. Spread 1 teaspoon Earth Balance on toast or enjoy dry.

*Snack:*

1 stalk celery cut into 3 pieces, with 1 tablespoon almond butter divided and spread evenly into each

## TUESDAY

*Breakfast:*

**POACHED ASPARAGUS
DELIGHT**

2 eggs
5 spears roasted asparagus
3 tablespoons thinly sliced red onion
2 tablespoons distilled vinegar

Preheat oven to 425°F. Lay asparagus out on a foil-lined baking sheet. Spray with olive oil spray and sprinkle salt and pepper. Roast for 8 to 10 minutes. Meanwhile, bring a pot of water to a rolling boil. Add vinegar. Turn down heat slightly, crack eggs, and slide into water one at a time. When asparagus is ready, take out and lay on plate nicely. Gently take eggs out of water with slotted spoon and lay on top of asparagus. Sprinkle red onion slices over and enjoy!

*Snack:*

5 sliced cucumber rounds with 2 pieces sodium-free turkey, pinch of black pepper, and 5 rice crackers

## WEDNESDAY

*Breakfast:*

**HEARTY OATMEAL**

¾ cup dry oatmeal
1 cup water
½ cup almond milk
3 tablespoons blueberries
3 tablespoons flax seeds
¼ teaspoon cinnamon (optional)

Add water and oatmeal to a microwave-safe bowl and heat for 1½ minutes. Carefully remove bowl, stir in cinnamon, and add almond milk to reach desired consistency. Top with blueberries and flaxseeds.

*Snack:*

Handful of mixed nuts (approx. 4 nuts each of raw almonds, raw cashews, raw pecans) with 1 small apple or small pear

# THURSDAY

## Breakfast:

### TURKEY EGG WHITE SCRAMBLE

5 egg whites

3 slices cooked turkey, chopped

4 tablespoons diced red pepper

½ cup fresh spinach

3 sliced fresh basil leaves

2 tablespoons finely diced leeks (white part only)

Pinch of black pepper

Starting with the leeks, add all ingredients to a pan except basil and turkey. When scramble is cooked (3 minutes), add turkey to warm it, place on plate, and sprinkle fresh basil on top.

## Snack:

½ banana sliced over ½ cup low-fat cottage cheese, sprinkled with 2 tablespoons slivered almonds

# FRIDAY

## Breakfast:

### BAKED EGGS

1 piece gluten-free bread

1 medium-sized ramekin

1 egg

2 egg whites

3 pieces chopped broccoli heads (no stems)

1 tablespoon finely diced shallots

2 halved cherry tomatoes

Place bread in toaster. Lightly spray ramekin with olive oil spray, add shallots, broccoli, and 2 halves of the cherry tomatoes. Add egg whites on top and crack egg over. Place the remaining halves of tomatoes on top. Back at 350°F for 15 minutes or until yolk is set. Sprinkle with salt and pepper.

## Snack:

Veggie plate: 3 cherry tomatoes, 3 baby carrots, 3 slices of green bell pepper, 3 tablespoons white bean hummus (white beans, lemon, olive oil, salt and pepper)

# SATURDAY

## Breakfast:

### COTTAGE CHEESE PARFAIT

1 cup low-fat cottage cheese

½ banana

6 raspberries

2 tablespoons sliced almonds

2 teaspoons hemp seeds

Place cottage cheese in a bowl. Place raspberries in a circle around cottage cheese; add sliced bananas in the same fashion in the middle of the raspberry circle. Top with almonds and sprinkle with hemp seeds.

## Snack:

15 protein pretzels dipped in 3 tablespoons cashew butter

# SUNDAY

## Breakfast:

### BAKED SPANISH EGGS

1 ramekin

1 egg

3 tablespoons diced canned tomatoes

1 teaspoon oregano

3 tablespoons chickpeas

1 piece gluten-free bread

Place bread in toaster. Spray ramekin lightly with olive oil, add tomatoes, chickpeas, and a pinch of oregano. Crack egg on top and sprinkle with salt and pepper. Bake at 350°F for 15 minutes or until yolk has set to your liking.

## Snack:

Homemade salsa: diced tomatoes, red onion, cilantro, small amount of jalapeño, minced clove fresh garlic, touch of olive oil, salt and pepper. Serve with 8 black bean chips.

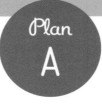

## Plan A

## Clean

### MONDAY

**TARRAGON TUNA SALAD**

2 cups shredded lettuce
¼ cup green pepper
¼ cup chopped cucumber
¼ cup diced tomatoes
1 teaspoon tarragon
3 ounces water-packed tuna

Place all ingredients into one bowl. Add a splash of balsamic vinegar and touch of extra virgin olive oil to salad. Mix together. Serve with 4 gluten-free crackers or rice crackers.

**Afternoon Snack:**

Hard-boiled egg with 5 small carrots and 5 rice crackers

### TUESDAY

Lunch:

**MEXICAN SHRIMP RICE BOWL**

¾ cup cooked brown rice
4 tablespoons black beans
½ cup diced tomatoes
¼ cup sliced chives
handful of fresh cilantro
6 whole cooked shrimp
Salt and pepper
Light drizzle of olive oil

To a hot pan, add 6 whole shrimp. Sauté for 1 minute each side. Add the rest of the ingredients and turn down to low. Heat through and enjoy!

**Afternoon Snack:**

Half of an avocado spread over one rice cake and 12 cashews

### WEDNESDAY

Lunch:

**CHICKEN SKEWER WITH WHITE BEAN HUMMUS**

1 3-ounce grilled chicken skewer
4 spears roasted asparagus
¾ cup cooked beluga lentils
¼ cup white bean hummus to dip

Sear chicken in skillet for 2 minutes on each side, or until there is no pink in the center and clear juices come out when sliced. Boil asparagus until tender, about 3 minutes. Cook lentils as directed on package. Puree white beans, olive oil, freshly squeezed lemon, and salt and pepper for hummus. Plate it and enjoy!

**Afternoon Snack:**

3 thick cucumber sticks wrapped with sodium-free turkey breast served with 1 tablespoon honey mustard to dip and 12 raw almonds

# THURSDAY

## Lunch:

### TURKEY LETTUCE CUPS

4 butter lettuce leaves
5 ounces cooked ground white-meat turkey or crumbled tempeh
2 tablespoons soy sauce
1 teaspoon sesame oil or olive oil
¼ cup diced carrots
Sprinkle of red chili flakes
¼ cup chopped fresh mint

Separate lettuce leaves and set aside. In a hot skillet, add olive oil, turkey or tempeh, carrots, and soy sauce. When cooked through, drizzle sesame oil on top and sprinkle with red chili flakes to your desired "hotness."

## Afternoon Snack:

2 slices lite Swiss cheese with 4 gluten-free rice crackers, served with handful of organic blueberries

# FRIDAY

## Lunch:

### CUMIN-DUSTED SALMON SALAD

4 ounces roast salmon dusted with cumin
2 cups arugula
½ cup chickpeas
5 halved cherry tomatoes
½ a fresh lemon
Salt and pepper

Add salmon to a medium high-heat pan with a touch of olive oil. Sprinkle with cumin, salt, and pepper. Flip carefully. When cooked all the way through (4 to 6 minutes), let cool slightly and flake the salmon over arugula, chickpeas, and cherry tomatoes. Squeeze lemon on top and add a pinch of salt and pepper.

## Afternoon Snack:

3 tablespoons edamame hummus dip (2 cups edamame or frozen edamame blanched, 2 tablespoons olive oil, fresh lemon, salt and pepper, pureed together) served with sliced bell pepper (6 slices total—3 from red, 3 from green) and 8 protein pretzels

# SATURDAY

## Lunch:

### HEARTY BUNLESS VEGGIE BURGER WITH ZUCCHINI FRIES

1 grilled veggie burger patty
3 tablespoons edamame hummus dip (see Friday's Afternoon Snack for recipe)
¼ cup arugula
½ avocado, sliced

Spread edamame hummus dip over patty. Top with arugula and avocado. Serve with grilled zucchini sticks (slice zucchini into ½-thick pieces, drizzle with olive oil, add salt and pepper, and place in hot pan to sear on all sides).

## Afternoon Snack:

2 baby dill pickles, 3 small cubes of white cheddar cheese, and 6 cashews

# SUNDAY

## Lunch:

### VEGETABLE QUINOA SALAD WITH FRESH HERBS AND GRILLED CHICKEN

4 ounces grilled chicken breast
½ cup cooked quinoa
1 cup diced tomatoes
1 cup chickpeas
½ cup diced celery
¼ cup finely diced red onion
½ cup diced red pepper
5 large, thinly sliced basil leaves
5 large, thinly sliced mint leaves
¼ cup olive oil
3 tablespoons red wine vinegar
Salt and pepper

In a medium-sized bowl, add all of the ingredients except the chicken and stir well. Let the flavors meld for a few minutes while you cook chicken on the grill or over the stove until completely cooked through (about 4 to 6 minutes).

## Afternoon Snack:

½ cup Greek yogurt mixed with 6 raw pecans and ½ apple, diced with a sprinkling of ground cinnamon

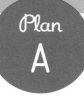

## Plan A

### Clean

<table>
<tr><th>MONDAY</th><th>TUESDAY</th><th>WEDNESDAY</th></tr>
</table>

**MONDAY**

*Dinner:*

**GRILLED LEMON TILAPIA, BROWN RICE, AND GREEN SALAD**

4 ounces fresh tilapia
½ cup cooked brown rice
1 teaspoon olive oil

GREEN SALAD:
2 cups spinach
¼ cup diced cucumber
¼ cup chopped tomatoes
2 tablespoons red wine vinegar
1 teaspoon Dijon mustard
3 tablespoons olive oil
Salt and pepper

Heat a grill pan on moderately high heat. Spray with olive oil and lay fish down gently. Squeeze half a lemon over fish and start to prepare salad. In a small bowl, whisk together dressing ingredients: red wine vinegar, mustard, oil, and salt and pepper. Set aside. Gently flip fish over and turn heat to low. Reheat brown rice, dress salad, and plate!

**TUESDAY**

*Dinner:*

**MEAT AND QUINOA**

4 ounces fillet mignon or favorite lean beef
½ cup cooked quinoa
5 spears roasted asparagus
5 steamed medium-sized carrots
a drizzle of balsamic vinegar

Heat a heavy cast-iron pan and spray with olive oil. Season beef on both sides with salt and pepper. When pan is hot, lay beef down. Do not move beef for 2 to 3 minutes. You want to get a nice sear. Meanwhile, trim asparagus and peel carrots. Spray lightly with olive oil, lay on sheet pan, and roast in oven for 15 minutes. (Option: For a more tender texture, parboil carrots for a few minutes before roasting.) Turn beef over after 2 to 3 minutes until beef is cooked to your liking. Reheat quinoa, and plate vegetables and beef. Drizzle with balsamic vinegar and enjoy!

**WEDNESDAY**

*Dinner:*

**FLAVOR-PACKED VEGETABLE CURRY**

½ cup cooked wheatberries
1 cup cauliflower
1 cup chickpeas
1 large carrot, diced
½ onion, diced
½ cup broccoli florets
2 cloves chopped garlic
3 tablespoons coconut oil
1 teaspoon curry powder
1 teaspoon garam masala
1 teaspoon turmeric
¼ teaspoon cayenne pepper
Salt and pepper

Add everything to a large skillet and sauté on medium heat until vegetables are golden; add drops of water if you find veggies are burning. Once colored, add 2 cups water or chicken stock, and cover for 10 minutes or until veggies are tender. Place over cooked wheatberries and sprinkle with sesame seeds.

# THURSDAY

## Dinner:

### KALE AND WHITE BEAN SOUP SERVED WITH GLUTEN-FREE BREAD

3 tablespoons olive oil

1 large onion diced

4 cloves chopped garlic

½ cup sliced cherry tomatoes

1 bunch kale, cleaned, veins removed, and chopped into bite-sized pieces

2 cups cannellini beans

1 slice gluten-free bread

Sauté onion, garlic, and tomatoes with olive oil for 3 minutes, then add kale and beans. Stir to coat for about 1 minute. Add 6 cups chicken or vegetable stock. Cover and let simmer for 40 minutes. Toast bread to desired doneness. Serve with chili flakes for garnish.

# FRIDAY

## Dinner:

### KICKED-UP TURKEY CHILI

⅓ cup chopped onion

1 diced green bell pepper

3 cloves chopped garlic

2 teaspoons cumin

2 teaspoons chili powder

1 teaspoon crushed pepper flakes

8 ounces ground white turkey meat

1 cup tomato sauce

¾ cup black beans

¾ cup kidney beans

Handful fresh cilantro

In a large, heavy pot, sauté onion, green bell pepper, garlic, cumin, chili powder, and crushed pepper flakes for 3 to 4 minutes. Add turkey until meat turns opaque (about 3 minutes). Add tomato sauce, black beans, kidney beans, and cilantro. Simmer on low for about 25 minutes. Eat as is, or serve with 4 gluten-free crackers.

# SATURDAY

## Dinner:

### ALMOND BUTTER KALE WITH LENTILS AND JUICY CHICKEN

½ cup beluga lentils

4 ounces chicken breast

3 cups kale, cleaned, veins removed, and chopped into bite-sized pieces

2 tablespoons almond butter

½ cup filtered water

1 teaspoon sesame seeds

Cook lentils as directed on package. Grill chicken on grill or in sauté pan for about 4 to 6 minutes, or until cooked through. Sauté kale with almond butter; add water to thin out sauce. Serve chicken on top of warm almond-kale mixture and lentils and sprinkle with sesame seeds.

# SUNDAY

## Dinner:

### TEMPEH BOWL WITH BROWN RICE TORTILLA FOR SCOOPING

4 ounces grilled tempeh

¼ cup chopped red onion

1 chopped carrot

½ cup black beans

¾ can diced tomatoes

¼ cup diced celery

3 cloves chopped garlic

½ finely diced jalapeño

1 teaspoon cumin

1 teaspoon coriander

Salt and pepper

Handful fresh parsley, chopped

2 small or one large rice-flour tortilla(s)

In large skillet, add all ingredients except tempeh, parsley, and tortillas. Sauté with 2 tablespoons olive oil until everything is tender. Should be rather soupy. Heat tortilla(s) in large skillet just to warm through. Serve in large shallow bowl with grilled tempeh. Garnish with parsley.

## DIET PLAN B: *Lean*

Since I have craved and adopted different ways of eating healthily at different times, I wanted to give you some options as well. For that reason, I asked Melissa Costello, creator of Karma Chow and personal chef to fitness guru Tony Horton, to offer a lacto-ovo meal plan geared toward wholesome foods that levels out blood-sugar levels. This diet is also a modified candida, or yeast-free, plan where carbs are essentially eliminated. I've had a lot of success following a low-carb diet, even with a meatless modification, since I am a nonmeat eater.

A high protein, no-sugar, low-carb option, this plan will give your body sustained energy, balanced blood sugar, and high nutrition. It will also allow your digestive system to recalibrate, give your body a much-needed break from sugars, and help bring it back into balance.

Since this option includes animal products such as cheese, eggs, and yogurt, Melissa recommends buying the highest quality available and know where they come from.

Remember, the key is to eat only whole foods, which means no processed foods. Why? You get the most energy and life out of foods that are still in their whole form. Make nuts and seeds your friend and take advantage of healthy fats, such as avocado and the high-quality oils that are included on the grocery list. You will eliminate starchy vegetables in this option, so stick to nonstarchy veggies (see grocery list), which will give you the energy and nutrients you need without the sugar highs and lows.

Grains and fruit are completely eliminated in this diet plan, since our goal is to provide you with optimal blood-sugar levels. Eating mainly veggies, nuts, seeds, healthy fats, and minimal amounts of animal proteins will do this.

Tofu is allowed, but use it in small amounts (once or twice per week), as it is processed. Tempeh is a great alternative, as it's fermented with whole grains, so it has live active cultures, which are great for digestion. It's loaded with protein and great for sustained energy.

You may find this option more challenging than the Clean option on page 242, but you may find that it suits your body to eliminate sugars. Results you can expect from following the Lean option include mental clarity, improved digestion, clearer skin, brighter eyes, better sleep, and sustained, balanced energy. Lastly, just a reminder: This plan does not restrict calories, so be very mindful of what your body needs versus what your mind wants, and eat accordingly. It's a process of starting to really tune in to listening to your body. I find that when I eliminate sugars, my cravings subside and my appetite levels out.

Check out the recipes and shopping list as a guideline on where you can begin.

## PLAN B: *Lean* GROCERY LIST

This is a general shopping list of all the foods you can eat on the Lean plan. Buying certain foods in bulk, such as nuts and grains, will save you money. Remember to stay away from packaged, processed foods.

### PROTEINS:
- [ ] Eggs
- [ ] Tempeh
- [ ] Tofu

### DAIRY:
- [ ] Goat or sheep's milk feta
- [ ] Goat cheese
- [ ] Goat's milk yogurt
- [ ] Greek yogurt
- [ ] Parmesan
- [ ] Plain, unsweetened, organic kefir

### NUTS & SEEDS (RAW ONLY):
- [ ] Almonds, cashews, hazelnuts, macadamias, pecans, pine nuts, pistachios, walnuts
- [ ] Chia seeds, flax seeds, pumpkin seeds, sesame seeds, sunflower seeds
- [ ] Raw nut and seed butters (no sugar added): almond, cashew, macadamia, pumpkin, sunflower, tahini

### GRAINS (EAT ONLY 3 TO 5 TIMES PER WEEK):
- [ ] Amaranth
- [ ] Buckwheat
- [ ] Millet
- [ ] Quinoa
- [ ] Wild rice

### OILS:
- [ ] Almond oil
- [ ] Avocado oil
- [ ] Coconut oil (extra-virgin, raw, unprocessed
- [ ] Flax oil
- [ ] Hazelnut oil
- [ ] Macadamia nut oil
- [ ] Olive oil (unfiltered, cold-pressed)
- [ ] Sesame oil (toasted and plain)
- [ ] Walnut oil

### NON-STARCHY VEGETABLES:
- [ ] Arugula
- [ ] Artichokes
- [ ] Asparagus
- [ ] Avocados
- [ ] Beet greens (tops)
- [ ] Bok choy
- [ ] Broccoli
- [ ] Brussels sprouts
- [ ] Burdock root
- [ ] Cabbage
- [ ] Cauliflower
- [ ] Celery
- [ ] Celery root
- [ ] Celeriac
- [ ] Collard greens
- [ ] Cucumbers
- [ ] Daikon radish
- [ ] Dandelion greens
- [ ] Eggplant
- [ ] Endive
- [ ] Escarole
- [ ] Fennel
- [ ] Garlic
- [ ] Ginger
- [ ] Jicama
- [ ] Kale
- [ ] Kohlrabi
- [ ] Leafy green lettuces
- [ ] Leeks
- [ ] Mushrooms
- [ ] Mustard greens
- [ ] Okra
- [ ] Olives
- [ ] Onions
- [ ] Radishes
- [ ] Radicchio
- [ ] Scallions
- [ ] Shallots
- [ ] Snow peas
- [ ] Spinach
- [ ] Sprouts
- [ ] Swiss chard
- [ ] Tomatoes
- [ ] Turnips
- [ ] Watercress
- [ ] Yellow squash
- [ ] Zucchini

### FRESH HERBS:
- [ ] Basil
- [ ] Chives
- [ ] Cilantro
- [ ] Dill
- [ ] Marjoram
- [ ] Oregano
- [ ] Parsley
- [ ] Thyme

### FRUITS:
- [ ] Green apple (Granny Smith)
- [ ] Lemons
- [ ] Limes
- [ ] White grapefruit

### CONDIMENTS:
- [ ] Apple cider vinegar (raw, unfiltered)
- [ ] Balsamic vinegar
- [ ] Bragg's Liquid Aminos (soy sauce substitute)
- [ ] Brown rice vinegar (unsweetened)
- [ ] Dijon mustard (stone-ground)
- [ ] Nama Shoyu (unpasteurized wheat-free soy sauce)
- [ ] Tamari (low-sodium, wheat-free soy sauce)

## Plan B

## Lean

# MONDAY

### Breakfast:

**VEGGIE EGG SCRAMBLE WITH AVOCADO AND TOMATO SLICES**

4 large eggs
2 tablespoons filtered water
Fresh chopped herbs of your choice
Dash cayenne
Sea salt and pepper, to taste
2 teaspoons coconut or olive oil
2 diced scallions, white parts only
½ diced red bell pepper
½ diced yellow bell pepper
5 stalks chopped asparagus
½ tomato, sliced
½ avocado, sliced

In a medium-sized bowl, beat eggs and water together with a wire whisk until well blended. Whisk in herbs, cayenne, sea salt, and pepper. In a nonstick skillet or cast-iron pan, heat coconut oil over medium heat and sauté scallions, peppers, and asparagus until soft but still crisp. Add eggs and let cook for a few minutes to start to harden, then continue stirring until eggs are set and firm. Do not overcook! Serve immediately with avocado and tomato slices.

### Snack:

**Handful of cashews**

# TUESDAY

### Breakfast:

**GREEK YOGURT WITH NUTS AND GREEN APPLE**

1 cup Greek yogurt, plain
1 tablespoon chopped nuts, your choice
½ green apple, diced

Place all ingredients in a small bowl and stir to combine.

### Snack:

**AVOCADO NUT SHAKE**

1 avocado, pitted and meat removed
½ cup almonds or cashews
2 cups water
1 teaspoon vanilla extract
4 drops stevia extract
Dash cinnamon
Dash nutmeg
Pinch sea salt
Handful ice (about 4 to 6 cubes)

Place all ingredients in a high-powered blender and blend until creamy smooth!

# WEDNESDAY

### Breakfast:

**VEGETABLE HERB FRITTATA**

4 large eggs
1 tablespoon freshly chopped dill
1 tablespoon freshly chopped basil
½ teaspoon dried oregano
¼ teaspoon sea salt
1 tablespoon coconut oil
1 thinly sliced small zucchini
½ thinly sliced cup mushrooms
½ cup finely chopped spinach
2 diced scallions, white parts only
1 tablespoon Parmesan cheese

Preheat oven to 400°F. Whisk eggs together in a large bowl with herbs and sea salt. Stir in remaining ingredients. Heat coconut oil in a cast-iron pan or nonstick oven-safe skillet over medium heat. Add scallions, mushrooms, and zucchini. Sauté until soft and slightly browned. Spread vegetables out evenly in bottom of pan and pour in egg mixture. Let cook for about 6 to 7 minutes or until bottom starts to harden. Top will still be runny. Sprinkle on Parmesan cheese evenly and transfer pan to oven and cook for about 5 to 8 minutes more, until top is set. Switch to broiler and let brown for about a minute until top is golden. Remove from broiler and let set for about 5 minutes.

### Snack:

**Celery with Nut Butter**

# THURSDAY

Breakfast:

## TOFU VEGGIE SCRAMBLE

1 tablespoon coconut oil

1 finely diced small red onion

1 clove minced garlic

½ cup thinly sliced mushrooms

1 diced red bell pepper

½ cup diced zucchini

¼ cup diced Roma tomatoes

1 pound extra-firm tofu, drained and crumbled

⅛ teaspoon turmeric

1 teaspoon cumin

3 tablespoons nutritional yeast

Heat coconut oil in a nonstick or cast-iron pan over medium heat. Add onion and garlic and sauté for a couple minutes or until softened. Add the mushrooms, pepper, zucchini, and tomatoes and cook until mushrooms are golden brown and pepper is soft. Add the crumbled tofu, spices, and nutritional yeast and stir well to incorporate. Cook for about 5 to 8 minutes more, stirring occasionally. Add small amounts of water if the tofu sticks. Season with salt and pepper to taste.

Snack:

**Handful of almonds**

# FRIDAY

Breakfast:

## SCRAMBLED EGGS WITH HERBS

2 large eggs and one egg white

2 teaspoons water or almond milk (unsweetened)

1 teaspoon coconut oil

2 teaspoons finely chopped fresh herbs of your choice (I love to use dill or basil)

Sea salt & freshly ground pepper to taste

Scramble eggs with water or almond milk in a medium bowl using a whisk. Whisk in herbs. Heat coconut oil on a skillet over medium heat. Add eggs and scramble until firm. Season with salt and pepper.

Snack:

**Greek Yogurt with Nuts and Cinnamon**

1 cup Greek yogurt, plain

1 tablespoon chopped nuts, your choice

½ teaspoon cinnamon

Place all ingredients in a small bowl and stir to combine.

# SATURDAY

Breakfast:

## MISO SOUP AND TEX MEX VEGGIE "SCRAMBLE"

2 tablespoons olive oil

1 diced green bell pepper

½ diced red bell pepper

10 thinly sliced mushrooms

1 finely minced shallot

1 teaspoon minced garlic

4 asparagus spears, cut into small pieces

1 teaspoon cumin

½ teaspoon coriander

1 teaspoon chili powder

1 tablespoon Bragg's Liquid Aminos

1 tablespoon water

½ cup halved cherry tomatoes

1 cup diced zucchini

½ cup diced yellow squash

3 tablespoons nutritional yeast

½ cup Swiss chard or kale, torn into small pieces

Heat the olive oil in a large, nonstick skillet over medium heat and sauté the peppers, mushrooms, shallots, and garlic until soft. Add the asparagus, cumin, chili powder, coriander, Bragg's, and water. Cover the skillet and let the asparagus steam until tender but still crisp, about 4 to 5 minutes. Add the tomatoes, zucchini, squash, and nutritional yeast and stir well to combine. Cook for another 5 minutes or until the veggies are soft but not mushy. Add the chard or kale and cover to wilt, about 3 minutes. Serve immediately.

Snack:

## AVOCADO NUT SHAKE

(See Tuesday's snack for recipe.)

# SUNDAY

Breakfast:

## SAVORY QUINOA BREAKFAST BOWL

1 cup quinoa, rinsed and drained, cooked according to package

½ cup shredded zucchini

Sesame seeds

Dulse flakes (optional)

DRESSING:

¼ cup tahini sauce

1 tablespoon Bragg's Liquid Aminos

1 tablespoon apple cider vinegar

1 tablespoon balsamic vinegar

Juice of 1 lemon

¼ cup filtered water

1 clove garlic

2 tablespoons olive oil

Place all sauce ingredients into a blender cup and blend until smooth and creamy. This will be a thick sauce, so feel free to add more water if you want it thinner.

Divide cooked quinoa and raw zucchini shreds into bowls, top with sauce, and sprinkle sesame seeds and dulse flakes on top.

Snack:

**Edamame and Celery Sticks**

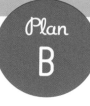

## Plan B

## Lean

### MONDAY

*Lunch:*

**PUMPKIN SEEDS AND ROASTED ASPARAGUS SOUP WITH KALE SALAD**

- 2 bunches fresh asparagus, chopped into 2-inch pieces
- 2 cloves minced garlic
- 3 stalks diced celery
- 1 thinly sliced leek, white parts only
- 1 diced small yellow onion
- 1 teaspoon dried tarragon
- 4 cups veggie broth
- 2 tablespoons olive oil
- ½ cup cashew cream (see recipe from Wednesday's dinner, page 256)

Preheat oven to 400°F. Toss asparagus with a drizzle of olive and place on a baking sheet in a single layer. Bake for about 20 minutes or until tender. In a large soup pot over medium heat, sauté garlic, celery, leek, and onion until soft. Add asparagus, tarragon, and veggie broth. Bring to a boil, reduce heat, and cover. Simmer for about 10 minutes. Remove from heat and puree with hand blender or regular blender (if using regular blender, let soup cool a bit first.) Pour soup back into pot and add cashew cream, stirring well to combine. Add sea salt and pepper to taste.

**KALE SALAD:**
(see page 265 for recipe.)

*Afternoon Snack:*

**Edamame**

### TUESDAY

*Lunch:*

**LEFTOVER GRILLED VEGGIES WITH TANGY AVOCADO CUCUMBER GAZPACHO**

- 2 peeled, chopped English cucumbers
- 1 ripe avocado
- 1 yellow bell pepper
- 1 teaspoon chopped jalapeño or ¼ teaspoon cayenne (optional)
- 2 chopped scallions
- ¼ cup fresh basil
- Juice of 1 lime
- ¼ cup water
- 2 tablespoons olive oil
- 2 teaspoons unsweetened rice vinegar

Place all ingredients except oil in blender and blend until smooth. While motor is running, slowly pour in oil. Blend until light and creamy. Add salt to taste. Serve chilled.

*Afternoon Snack:*

**SALSA & GUACAMOLE WITH CUCUMBERS**

- 3 avocados, pitted and skins removed
- ¼ cup finely diced shallots
- 10 quartered cherry tomatoes
- ½ seeded and minced jalapeño (optional)
- 3 tablespoons freshly squeezed lime juice
- Sea salt and pepper, to taste
- Fresh cilantro (optional)

Gently mash avocadoes in a medium sized bowl, leaving some chunks. Add remaining ingredients and stir well to combine. If refrigerating, place pits on top of guacamole to prevent browning. Cover and chill.

### WEDNESDAY

*Lunch:*

**THAI CUCUMBER SALAD AND LEFTOVER ASPARAGUS SOUP**

- 1 English cucumber, halved lengthwise and cut into ¼-inch half rounds
- ½ yellow or red bell pepper, finely diced
- 2 scallions, finely chopped
- Handful fresh basil, chopped
- ¼ cup cashews, chopped

DRESSING:
- Juice of 1 lime
- 1 clove minced garlic
- 1 tablespoon Bragg's Liquid Aminos
- 1 tablespoon rice vinegar
- 2 tablespoons sesame oil
- 1 tablespoon water
- Pinch red pepper flakes
- 2 to 4 drops stevia extract, to taste

Whisk dressing ingredients together in a small bowl.

Place all salad ingredients in a medium-sized bowl. Pour dressing over and stir well to combine. Heat soup and enjoy together!

*Afternoon Snack:*

**GREEK YOGURT WITH NUTS AND NUTMEG**

- 1 cup Greek yogurt, plain
- 1 tablespoon chopped nuts, your choice
- ½ teaspoon nutmeg

Place all ingredients in a small bowl and stir to combine.

# THURSDAY

## Lunch:

### LEFTOVER CAULIFLOWER SOUP AND ASIAN SLAW

1 head thinly sliced Napa cabbage
1 julienned red bell pepper
1 cup julienned snow peas
1 thinly sliced shallot

DRESSING:

2 tablespoons rice vinegar
1 tablespoon lime juice
2 tablespoons toasted sesame oil
3 drops stevia extract
Dash crushed red pepper flakes

Place all dressing ingredients in blender and blend until combined. Pour over cabbage mixture and refrigerate for 1 hour to let flavors meld.

## Afternoon Snack:

### SUNFLOWER SEED DIP WITH JICAMA SLICES

2 cup sunflower seeds, soaked for 4 hours
1 roasted yellow bell pepper
¼ chopped jalapeño
1 handful fresh parsley
1 handful fresh basil
1 tablespoon apple cider vinegar
2 tablespoons lemon juice
1 clove garlic
1 tablespoon Bragg's Liquid Aminos
2 to 4 tablespoons olive oil, depending on creaminess

Place all ingredients in a food processor except the olive oil. Puree together, scraping sides occasionally. While motor is running pour olive oil in the top and puree until smooth.

# FRIDAY

## Lunch:

### WARM ASPARAGUS AND ARTICHOKE SALAD WITH CURRIED CAULIFLOWER

1 tablespoon olive oil
½ diced yellow onion
3 thinly sliced shiitake mushrooms
1 bunch asparagus, cut into 1-inch pieces
1 can artichoke hearts, drained, rinsed, and roughly chopped
4 sundried tomatoes, soaked and cut into small strips
15 black olives, halved
1 teaspoon thyme
2 tablespoons balsamic vinegar
2 tablespoons water
1 tablespoon goat cheese, crumbled

Heat olive oil in skillet over medium heat and sauté onion and mushrooms together. Add artichoke hearts, asparagus, sundried tomatoes, olives, thyme, balsamic vinegar, and water. Cover with lid and cook for about 5 to 7 minutes or until asparagus is tender and artichoke hearts are warmed through. Top with crumbled goat cheese and serve warm.

### CURRIED CAULIFLOWER:

(For ingredients and instructions, see Monday's dinner recipe, page 256.)

## Afternoon Snack:

Caprese Salad with Goat Cheese (in place of mozzarella)

# SATURDAY

## Lunch:

### LEFTOVER TEMPEH WITH JICAMA SLAW

1 jicama, peeled and julienned
1 grated green apple, with skin
½ sliced small red onion
1 red bell pepper, thinly sliced

DRESSING:

Juice of 1 lime
2 tablespoons olive oil
2 tablespoons apple cider vinegar
4 drops stevia extract
½ teaspoon red chili flakes
1 tablespoon chopped cilantro
½ cubed avocado (as garnish)

Place ingredients in large bowl. Whisk together dressing ingredients and pour over slaw. Toss to incorporate and top with avocado.

## Afternoon Snack:

### CELERY AND GUACAMOLE

3 avocados, pitted and meat removed
¼ cup finely diced shallots
10 quartered cherry tomatoes
3 tablespoons fresh lime juice
Sea salt and pepper, to taste
½ jalapeño, seeded and minced (optional)
Fresh cilantro (optional)

Gently mash avocados in a medium-sized bowl, leaving some chunks. Add remaining ingredients and stir well to combine. If refrigerating, place pits on top of guacamole to prevent browning. Cover and chill.

# SUNDAY

## Lunch:

### LEFTOVER KABOBS AND SIDE SALAD

See Saturday's dinner, page 257. Enjoy a small green salad of your choice.

## Afternoon Snack:

### AVOCADO NUT SHAKE

1 avocado, pitted and meat removed
½ cup almonds or cashews
2 cups water
1 teaspoon vanilla extract
4 drops stevia extract
Dash cinnamon
Dash nutmeg
Pinch sea salt
Handful ice (about 4 to 6 cubes)

Place all ingredients in a high-powered blender and blend until creamy smooth!

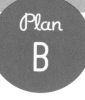

## Plan B

### Lean

# MONDAY

**Dinner:**

## GRILLED VEGGIE MEDLEY WITH CURRIED CAULIFLOWER

2 tablespoons olive oil

3 tablespoons balsamic vinegar

3 tablespoons water

1 tablespoon Dijon mustard

Fresh dried herbs (oregano, basil, thyme, etc.)

**USE ANY COMBINATION OF THE FOLLOWING VEGGIES:**

Eggplant, zucchini, red onion, yellow squash, tomatoes (leave whole), mushroom, asparagus (trim ends, but leave stalk whole), bell peppers (leave whole and roast alone)

Cut veggies into ¼-inch-thick slices. Mix marinade ingredients and pour over veggies in a casserole dish. Let sit for 20 minutes. Preheat grill and roast veggies until tender, flipping once or twice to prevent burning. Enjoy!

**CURRIED CAULIFLOWER:**

1 tablespoon coconut oil

½ diced small yellow onion

2 cloves minced garlic

1 teaspoon cumin seeds

1 medium head of cauliflower, cut into 1-inch florets

1 tablespoon curry powder

1 teaspoon ginger powder

Juice of 1 lemon

1 cup water

½ teaspoon sea salt

In a large skillet with a tight-fitting lid, melt coconut oil over medium heat. Sauté onion, garlic, and cumin seeds until onion softens and cumin seeds start to brown. Add cauliflower, curry powder, ginger powder, lemon juice, water, and sea salt. Stir well to coat cauliflower with seasonings. Cover with lid, turn to low, and simmer until cauliflower is tender.

# TUESDAY

**Dinner:**

## STIR-FRY VEGGIES WITH TOFU & KALE SALAD

1 package firm tofu, drained and cubed

6 cups chopped veggies (use any combination of allowable veggies)

2 tablespoons of toasted sesame oil

Sesame seeds

Fresh chopped herbs

Heat sesame oil in a wok over medium heat and stir-fry tofu until brown. Add veggies and stir-fry until tender but still crisp and bright in color. Season with Bragg's Liquid Aminos or use the teriyaki sauce from the Tofu Kabob recipe included under Saturday's dinner. Top with sesame seeds and your choice of fresh herbs.

**KALE SALAD:**

**(See page 265 for recipe.)**

# WEDNESDAY

**Dinner:**

## CREAMY DILLED CAULIFLOWER SOUP WITH MIXED GREEN SALAD

2 tablespoons coconut or olive oil

3 stalks celery

1 diced medium yellow onion

2 cloves minced garlic

1 minced shallot

1 large head of cauliflower, cut into 1-inch florets

1 turnip, peeled and cut into ½-inch cubes

3 tablespoons freshly chopped dill (or 2 teaspoons of dried dill)

4 cups veggie broth

¼ cup cashew cream

Heat oil in soup pot over medium heat and sauté celery, onion, garlic, and shallot until soft and somewhat caramelized. Add cauliflower, turnip, dill, and veggie broth. Cover pot and bring to a boil over high heat. Once boiling, simmer for about 20 minutes or until cauliflower is soft. Puree soup using a hand blender or regular blender. Pour back in pot and stir in cashew cream. Salt and pepper to taste. Enjoy with large salad of your choice.

**CASHEW CREAM:**

1 cup cashews, soaked for 4 hours

½ to 1 cup coconut water

¼ cup maple syrup or 4 drops Stevia

1 teaspoon vanilla extract

Put all ingredients in a blender and blend until smooth. If too thick, add more coconut water. Feel free to add cinnamon, nutmeg, or other spices.

# THURSDAY

## Dinner:

### COCONUT BASIL STIR-FRY WITH MIXED GREEN SALAD

**COCONUT SAUCE:**

1 cup chopped fresh basil leaves
1 cup regular coconut milk
1 tablespoon Bragg's Liquid Aminos
1 tablespoon fresh lemon juice
1 teaspoon minced fresh ginger
2 drops of stevia

**STIR-FRY:**

1 tablespoon coconut oil
2 cloves minced garlic
1 teaspoon fresh grated ginger
1 thinly sliced small red onion
1 cup broccoli florets
1 red bell pepper, cut into strips
1 cup thinly sliced mushrooms
1 cup thinly sliced bok choy or cabbage

Place all sauce ingredients in a blender and blend to combine.

In a large wok or sauté pan, heat coconut oil over medium-high heat. Sauté garlic and onion until translucent. Add ginger and sauté for another minute. Add red pepper and mushrooms. Cook for another 3 minutes. Add broccoli, bok choy, and coconut sauce. Cover with lid, reduce heat to medium, and let vegetables steam in the sauce for a few minutes. Stir occasionally. Do not overcook the vegetables or let them get soggy. Enjoy with large mixed green salad of your choice.

# FRIDAY

## Dinner:

### MARINATED TEMPEH WITH GRILLED VEGGIE MEDLEY

1 8-ounce package tempeh, divided into 4 triangles
3 tablespoons apple cider vinegar
¼ cup Bragg's Liquid Aminos
1 clove crushed garlic
2 tablespoons olive oil
1 tablespoon tomato paste
3 drops pure stevia liquid
1 teaspoon sesame seeds

Place cut tempeh in a baking dish in a single layer. Whisk marinade ingredients together and pour over tempeh. Let sit for about 20 minutes. Preheat oven to 350°F and bake for about 15 minutes. Turn tempeh and then bake for 10 more minutes. Remove from oven and serve with Balsamic Grilled Veggie Medley.

**GRILLED VEGGIE MEDLEY:**
(See Monday's dinner for recipe.)

# SATURDAY

## Dinner:

### TERIYAKI TOFU KABOBS WITH LARGE SPINACH SALAD

1 package extra-firm tofu, cut into 1-inch cubes
1 zucchini, cut into ½ inch pieces
1 yellow squash, cut into ½ inch pieces
1 red onion, cut into wedges
1 green bell pepper, cut into 1 inch pieces

**TERIYAKI SAUCE:**

¼ cup Bragg's Liquid Aminos
1 tablespoon balsamic vinegar
3 tablespoons rice vinegar
4 drops pure stevia extract
1 inch piece fresh ginger, grated
3 cloves minced garlic
1 tablespoon sesame oil

Blend all ingredients together in a blender until well combined. Pour over tofu and let marinate for 20 to 40 minutes in the refrigerator. While tofu is marinating, soak bamboo skewers (about 10) in water. Preheat grill. Take tofu out of fridge (save marinade) and thread it onto the soaked skewers, alternating with veggies. Put the kabobs in a large casserole dish and pour the leftover marinade on top. Place kabobs on the grill and let them cook, turning so that each side gets brown. Brush skewers with leftover marinade as they cook.

# SUNDAY

## Dinner:

### VEGGIE FAJITAS WITH SIDE SALAD (OPTIONAL QUINOA)

1 tablespoon olive oil
½ large yellow onion, thinly sliced
1 large portobello mushroom, thinly sliced
½ red bell pepper, thinly sliced
½ yellow bell pepper, thinly sliced
½ large zucchini or yellow squash, cut into ½-inch strips
3 Roma tomatoes, chopped small
1 teaspoon cumin
½ teaspoon oregano
2 teaspoons chili powder
Juice of 1 lime
1 tablespoon Bragg's Liquid Aminos
2 tablespoons chopped cilantro
Sea salt
Salsa and guacamole (optional)

Heat the olive oil in a large skillet over medium heat and sauté the onion and mushrooms. Cook for a few minutes until the onions are soft and the mushrooms have released their juices. Add the bell peppers, squash, tomatoes, cumin, oregano, chili powder, lime juice, Bragg's, and cilantro. Stir well to incorporate. Cover the skillet to let the veggies steam for about 5 to 7 minutes, stirring occasionally. Remove from heat and serve immediately with fresh salsa and guacamole. Enjoy with side salad of your choice or quinoa.

## DIET PLAN C: *Green*

Although I am not a strict vegan, I do have periods in my life when I am. Since I was raised a vegan macrobiotic (from age nine to eighteen), I do have those tendencies. Moreover I know how beneficial eating vegan can be and how good it feels. To craft this green plan, I asked vegan culinary expert Melissa Costello, creator of Karma Chow, to design a menu especially for people who would like to try it but don't know how to start. Even if you're a committed carnivore, you might enjoy trying it out!

This option is completely vegan, which means you will not be eating any animal products at all. Although that may sound scary or boring to you, I think you will find this option to be surprisingly satisfying. You will get to eat tons of fresh veggies, fruits, grains, nuts, seeds, and legumes. I've provided enough delicious and nutritious recipes that you won't even miss the meat in your life.

Melissa says, "In the past few years, veganism has often been thought of as a fad, or only a diet that animal activists followed, but this way of eating is making its way more and more into the American mainstream and people are gravitating to it in the quest for optimal health, weight loss, and energy. Big celebrities are now adopting this lifestyle as a way to become more vibrant and healthy while changing their relationship to food. And although this may seem a bit trendy, this way of eating truly is transformative."

One thing you may be thinking is, "What about protein? Where will I get my protein?" The answer is easy—from veggies, beans, grains, nuts, seeds, and fruits! Yes, there is protein in all of these options. It may not be the same amount of protein you are used to seeing or getting, but it's actually more bioavailable to the body and easier to digest and assimilate than animal-based protein.

The Green option also provides tons of variety and flavor as well as sustained energy. Some of the positive results you may feel are a lighter feeling in your body, clear thinking, stellar digestion, balanced blood sugar, and sustained energy. You may also feel less stressed and agitated because your energy is high and digestion is working like a well-oiled machine.

Out of all the plans, this one actually offers the most variety, and as a result, you may find it easy to integrate it into your everyday lifestyle versus a diet that you follow short-term.

# PLAN C: *Green* GROCERY LIST

This is a general shopping list of all the foods you can eat on the Green plan. Buying certain foods, such as nuts, beans, and grains, in bulk will save you money. Remember to stay away from packaged, processed foods.

## MEAT ALTERNATIVES:
- ☐ Tempeh
- ☐ Tofu

## UNSWEETENED DAIRY ALTERNATIVES:
- ☐ Almond milk
- ☐ Coconut milk
- ☐ Rice milk

## NUTS & SEEDS (RAW ONLY):
- ☐ Almonds, cashews, hazelnuts, macadamias, pecans, pine nuts, pistachios, walnuts
- ☐ Chia seeds, flax seeds, pumpkin seeds, sesame seeds, sunflower seeds
- ☐ Raw nut and seed butters (no sugar added): almond, cashew, macadamia, pumpkin, sunflower, tahini

## GRAINS:
- ☐ Amaranth
- ☐ Brown rice, both short- and long-grain
- ☐ Buckwheat
- ☐ Millet
- ☐ Quinoa
- ☐ Wild Rice

## OILS:
- ☐ Almond oil
- ☐ Avocado oil
- ☐ Coconut oil (extra-virgin, raw, unprocessed
- ☐ Flax oil
- ☐ Hazelnut oil
- ☐ Macadamia nut oil
- ☐ Olive oil (unfiltered, cold-pressed)
- ☐ Sesame oil (toasted and plain)
- ☐ Walnut oil

## VEGETABLES:
- ☐ Arugula
- ☐ Artichokes
- ☐ Asparagus
- ☐ Avocados
- ☐ Beet greens (tops)
- ☐ Beets
- ☐ Bok choy
- ☐ Broccoli
- ☐ Brussels sprouts
- ☐ Burdock root
- ☐ Butternut squash
- ☐ Cabbage
- ☐ Cauliflower
- ☐ Celery
- ☐ Celery root
- ☐ Celeriac
- ☐ Collard greens
- ☐ Corn
- ☐ Cucumbers
- ☐ Daikon radish
- ☐ Dandelion greens
- ☐ Endive
- ☐ Escarole
- ☐ Fennel
- ☐ Garlic
- ☐ Ginger
- ☐ Jicama
- ☐ Kabocha squash
- ☐ Kale
- ☐ Kohlrabi
- ☐ Leafy green lettuces
- ☐ Leeks
- ☐ Mushrooms
- ☐ Mustard greens
- ☐ Okra
- ☐ Olives
- ☐ Onions
- ☐ Peas
- ☐ Radishes
- ☐ Radicchio
- ☐ Red and purple potatoes
- ☐ Scallions
- ☐ Seaweed
- ☐ Shallots
- ☐ Snow peas
- ☐ Spinach
- ☐ Sprouts
- ☐ Sweet potatoes
- ☐ Swiss chard
- ☐ Tomatoes
- ☐ Turnips
- ☐ Watercress
- ☐ Garnet yams
- ☐ Yellow wquash
- ☐ Zucchini

## FRESH HERBS:
- ☐ Basil
- ☐ Chives
- ☐ Cilantro
- ☐ Dill
- ☐ Parsley
- ☐ Thyme
- ☐ Marjoram
- ☐ Oregano

## LEGUMES:
- ☐ Adzuki beans
- ☐ Black beans
- ☐ Chickpeas/Garbanzo beans
- ☐ Kidney beans
- ☐ Lentils
- ☐ Split Peas, yellow and green
- ☐ White beans

## FRUITS:
- ☐ Apples, any variety (Granny Smith has lowest sugar)
- ☐ Berries
- ☐ Grapefruit
- ☐ Lemons
- ☐ Limes
- ☐ Melon
- ☐ Pears
- ☐ Peaches
- ☐ Plums

## CONDIMENTS:
- ☐ Apple cider vinegar (raw, unfiltered)
- ☐ Balsamic vinegar
- ☐ Bragg's Liquid Aminos (soy sauce substitute)
- ☐ Brown rice vinegar (unsweetened)
- ☐ Dijon mustard (stone-ground)
- ☐ Nama Shoyu (unpasteurized wheat-free soy sauce)
- ☐ Tamari (low-sodium, wheat-free soy sauce)

# MONDAY

## Breakfast:

### MILLET WITH BERRIES, ALMOND MILK, AND NUTS

1 cup cooked millet
¼ cup fresh berries
¼ cup green apple, diced
Dash cinnamon
Dash cardamom
Dash nutmeg
1 to 2 tablespoons almond milk or coconut milk (unsweetened)
2 to 4 drops stevia extract
1 tablespoon shredded coconut
1 tablespoon nuts of your choice

## Snack:

1 apple with 1 tablespoon nut butter

# TUESDAY

## Breakfast:

### GREEN JUICE AND GINGERY MISO SOUP

1 cucumber
6 stalks celery
2 handfuls spinach
1 green apple
1 inch piece of ginger (optional)

Juice all ingredients together. Be sure to add spinach in the middle of the juicing process and add some celery afterward.

### GINGERY MISO SOUP:

4 cups water
1 tablespoon wakame seaweed, chopped into small pieces
2 teaspoons freshly grated ginger
2 thinly sliced shiitake mushrooms
1 thinly sliced green onion
3 tablespoons miso paste

In a saucepan, bring water, wakame, ginger, and green onion to a boil. Reduce heat and simmer for about 5 to 7 minutes. Remove from heat. In a small dish or cup, mix miso paste with about 3 tablespoons of water to make a thin paste. Add this to the pot and stir well to incorporate. Do NOT BOIL miso! Serve immediately.

## Snack:

One handful each of almonds and berries

# WEDNESDAY

## Breakfast:

### AVOCADO NUT SHAKE

1 avocado, pitted and meat removed
½ cup almonds or cashews
2 cups water
1 teaspoon vanilla extract
4 drops stevia extract
Dash cinnamon
Dash nutmeg
Pinch sea salt
Handful ice (about 4 to 6 cubes)

Place all ingredients in a high-powered blender and blend until creamy smooth

## Snack:

### BLACK BEAN DIP AND VEGGIES

2 cups black beans
½ jalapeño, deseeded and minced
1 red bell pepper, diced
½ red onion, diced
1 clove minced garlic
¼ teaspoon chipotle chili powder
1 teaspoon cumin
3 tablespoons olive oil
1 tablespoon apple cider vinegar
2 teaspoons maple syrup
½ teaspoon sea salt

In a skillet over medium heat, sauté jalapeño, bell pepper, onion, and garlic in 1 tablespoon olive oil until soft. Stir in cumin and chili powder. Remove from heat when ingredients are soft and caramelized. Place black beans, onion sauté, vinegar, and maple syrup in a food processor cup. Puree ingredients together, adding remaining olive oil while it's running. Scrape sides and puree again. Serve warm or chilled.

Serve with chopped fresh veggies of your choice (see Saturday snack).

# THURSDAY

## Breakfast:

### MILLET WITH ALMOND MILK AND BERRIES

1 cup cooked millet

¼ cup fresh berries

¼ cup green apple, diced

Dash cinnamon

Dash cardamom

Dash nutmeg

1 to 2 tablespoons almond milk or coconut milk (unsweetened)

2 to 4 drops stevia extract

1 tablespoon shredded coconut

1 tablespoon nuts of your choice

## Snack:

### GREEN JUICE

1 cucumber

6 stalks celery

2 handfuls spinach

1 green apple

1 inch piece of ginger (optional)

Juice all ingredients together. Be sure to add spinach in the middle of the juicing process and add some celery afterward.

# FRIDAY

## Breakfast:

### QUINOA BREAKFAST BOWL WITH FRESH FRUIT

1 cup cooked quinoa

¼ cup fresh berries

¼ cup green apple, diced

Dash cinnamon

Dash cardamom

Dash nutmeg

1 to 2 tablespoons almond milk or coconut milk (unsweetened)

2 to 4 drops stevia extract

1 tablespoon shredded coconut

1 tablespoon nuts of your choice

## Snack:

### CREAMY BERRY PROTEIN SHAKE

1 cup almond milk

1 scoop vanilla vegan protein powder

½ cup frozen berries

1 tablespoon raw almond or cashew butter

2 to 4 drops stevia extract

Handful of fresh spinach

Ice (optional)

Place all the ingredients in a high-powered blender and blend until creamy smooth!

# SATURDAY

## Breakfast:

### STEEL-CUT OATS WITH BERRIES, ALMOND MILK, AND NUTS

(See Monday's breakfast for recipe.)

## Snack:

### SPICY EDAMAME DIP AND VEGGIES

1 16-ounce package frozen, shelled edamame, cooked according to instructions and drained, or fresh edamame

4 cloves garlic

1¼ teaspoons sea salt

½ teaspoon ground coriander

½ teaspoon ground cumin

¼ teaspoon cayenne pepper

4 to 6 tablespoons olive oil

¼ cup fresh lime juice

¼ cup fresh cilantro

Place all ingredients except olive oil and lime juice into a food processor. Puree until combined. Add olive oil and lime juice and puree more, scraping sides of the processor bowl frequently. If you like a smoother consistency, add purified water, 1 tablespoon at a time, until desired texture is reached.

Serve with 1 cup of freshly chopped veggies, such as carrot sticks, celery sticks, cucumber slices, or jicama slices.

# SUNDAY

## Breakfast:

### TEMPEH VEGGIE SCRAMBLE

1 tablespoon of coconut oil

1 finely diced small red onion

1 clove minced garlic

½ cup thinly sliced mushrooms

1 diced red bell pepper

½ cup diced zucchini

¼ cup diced Roma tomatoes

1 8-ounce package tempeh, crumbled

⅛ teaspoon turmeric

1 teaspoon cumin

3 tablespoons nutritional yeast

Sea salt and ground pepper, to taste

Heat coconut oil in a nonstick or cast-iron pan over medium heat. Add onion and garlic and sauté for a couple minutes or until softened. Add the mushrooms, pepper, zucchini, and tomatoes and cook until mushrooms are golden brown and pepper is soft. Add the crumbled tempeh, spices, and nutritional yeast and stir well to incorporate. Cook for about 5 to 8 minutes more, stirring occasionally. Add small amounts of water if the tempeh begins to stick. Season with salt and pepper to taste.

## Snack:

1 green apple with 1 tablespoon nut butter

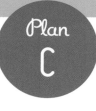

## Plan C

## Green

### MONDAY

*Lunch:*

**DILLED CARROT SOUP AND LARGE GREEN SALAD WITH VEGGIES**

2 tablespoons olive oil
1 diced yellow onion
3 cloves minced garlic
3 stalks diced celery
2 lbs carrots, peeled and cut into chunks
4 cups vegetable broth
2 tablespoons chopped fresh dill
½ cup coconut milk
1 teaspoon sea salt

In a large stockpot over medium heat, sauté onion, garlic, and celery in olive oil until soft. Add carrots, vegetable stock, and salt. Turn heat to high, cover pot and bring to a boil. Once boiling, turn down to a simmer and cook for about 20 minutes or until carrots are very soft. Remove from heat and puree using a hand blender. Add fresh dill and coconut milk and stir well to combine. Season with black pepper to taste.

*Afternoon Snack:*

**"CHEEZY" POPCORN**

1 tablespoon extra virgin coconut oil
½ cup organic corn kernels
Nutritional yeast flakes, to taste

In a large pot with a fitted lid, heat the coconut oil over medium heat until melted. Add popcorn kernels and cover. Wait until first kernel pops, then lower heat a tad. Popcorn will continue to pop; you do not need to shake the pot, but you can. Cook until you hear the popping slow.

Season with salt, pepper (optional), and nutritional yeast flakes for a "cheesy" flavor, and mix well or shake in a bag!

### TUESDAY

*Lunch:*

**LEFTOVER STIR-FRY VEGGIES AND SIDE SALAD**

(Reheat leftover stir-fry from Monday night's dinner. Serve with side salad and dressing of your choice.)

*Afternoon Snack:*

**BLACK BEAN DIP AND VEGGIES**

2 cup black beans
½ jalapeño, deseeded and minced
1 red bell pepper, diced
½ red onion, diced
1 clove minced garlic
¼ teaspoon chipotle chili powder
1 teaspoon cumin
3 tablespoons olive oil
1 tablespoon apple cider vinegar
2 teaspoons maple syrup
½ teaspoon sea salt

In a skillet over medium heat, sauté jalapeño, red bell pepper, onion, and garlic in 1 tablespoon olive oil until soft. Add cumin and chili powder and stir while cooking to incorporate. Remove from heat when all ingredients are soft and somewhat caramelized.

Place black beans, onion mixture, apple cider vinegar & maple syrup in a food processor cup. Puree ingredients together while pouring the remaining 2 tablespoons of olive oil in top of processor while running. Make sure you remove lid and scrape sides and puree again. Serve warm or chilled.

### WEDNESDAY

*Lunch:*

**LARGE GREEN SALAD WITH VEGGIE BURGER**

1 15-ounce can chickpeas or 1½ cups cooked
1 cup cooked brown rice
½ red bell pepper, cut into chunks
½ onion, cut into chunks
1 cup baby spinach
Handful fresh cilantro
1½ cups gluten-free breadcrumbs
2 tablespoons tomato paste
½ teaspoon chili powder
Sea salt and pepper, to taste

In food processor, pulse chickpeas and brown rice together about 10 times. Scrape into large bowl. Puree bell pepper, onion, cilantro, and spinach until well combined; this mixture will be very wet. Transfer the mixture into the bowl with the chickpea mixture. Stir in the breadcrumbs, tomato paste, chili powder, salt, and pepper. Mix with hands or wooden spoon to combine all ingredients. Form mixture into patties and heat on a grill or skillet with olive oil until golden brown. Serve with large green salad.

*Afternoon Snack:*

**CUP OF DILLED CARROT SOUP**

(Reheat leftovers from Monday's lunch.)

# THURSDAY

## Lunch:

### LEFTOVER WHITE BEAN AND SWEET POTATO SOUP AND TEMPEH "TUNA" SALAD

- 1 8-ounce package tempeh
- ½ finely diced small red onion
- 1 stalk finely diced celery
- 1 shredded carrot
- 2 tablespoons chopped dill pickles
- 1 tablespoon capers
- 1 tablespoon fresh, chopped dill
- 2 tablespoons grapeseed Vegenaise
- 1 teaspoon apple-cider vinegar
- Sea salt and pepper, to taste
- 1 cup White Bean and Sweet Potato Soup (see Wednesday's dinner)

Cut tempeh cubes and steam for about 7 minutes. (This helps to soften and remove the bitterness.) Remove and cool. Crumble tempeh into small pieces into a bowl. Add remaining ingredients and stir to combine. Serve chilled on a bed of baby greens or arugula. Reheat soup and enjoy!

## Afternoon Snack:

### AVOCADO NUT SHAKE

- 1 avocado, pitted and meat removed
- ½ cup almonds or cashews
- 2 cups water
- 1 teaspoon vanilla extract
- 4 drops stevia extract
- Dash cinnamon
- Dash nutmeg
- Pinch sea salt
- Handful ice (about 4 to 6 cubes)

Place all ingredients in a high-powered blender and blend until creamy smooth!

# FRIDAY

## Lunch:

### LARGE GREEN SALAD WITH TEMPEH "TUNA"

- 1 8-ounce package tempeh
- ½ finely diced small red onion
- 1 stalk finely diced celery
- 1 shredded carrot
- 2 tablespoons chopped dill pickles
- 1 tablespoon capers
- 1 tablespoon fresh, chopped dill
- 2 tablespoons grapeseed Vegenaise
- 1 teaspoon apple cider vinegar

Cut tempeh cubes and steam for about 7 minutes. Remove and cool. Crumble tempeh into small pieces into a bowl. Add remaining ingredients and stir to combine. Serve chilled on a bed of baby greens or arugula.

## Afternoon Snack:

### SPICY EDAMAME DIP AND VEGGIES

- 1 16-ounce package frozen, shelled edamame, cooked according to instructions and drained, or fresh edamame
- 4 cloves garlic
- 1¼ teaspoons sea salt
- ½ teaspoon ground coriander
- ½ teaspoon ground cumin
- ¼ teaspoon cayenne pepper
- 4 to 6 tablespoons olive oil
- ¼ cup fresh lime juice
- ¼ cup fresh cilantro

Puree all ingredients except olive oil and lime juice in a food processor. Add olive oil and lime juice and puree more, scraping sides of the bowl frequently. If you like a smoother consistency, add water, 1 tablespoon at a time, until desired texture is reached.

Serve with sliced freshed veggies of your choice.

# SATURDAY

## Lunch:

### LEFTOVER BLACK BEAN SWEET POTATO CHILI AND JICAMA SLAW

- 1 jicama, peeled and julienned
- 1 grated green apple, with skin
- ½ small red onion, thinly sliced
- 1 red bell pepper, thinly sliced
- Juice of 1 lime
- 2 tablespoons olive oil
- 2 tablespoons apple cider vinegar
- 4 drops stevia extract
- ½ teaspoon red chili flakes
- 1 tablespoon chopped cilantro
- ½ cubed avocado
- 1 cup Black Bean Sweet Potato Chili (see Friday's dinner)
- 1 cup Jicama Slaw (see page 255)

Place all ingredients in a large bowl. Whisk together dressing ingredients and pour over slaw to coat. Toss to incorporate, and top with cubed avocado. Reheat chili and enjoy!

## Afternoon Snack:

### GUACAMOLE WITH FRESH VEGGIES

- 3 avocados, pitted and meat removed
- ¼ cup finely diced shallot
- 10 quartered cherry tomatoes
- 3 tablespoons fresh lime juice
- ½ jalapeño, seeded and minced (optional)
- Fresh cilantro (optional)

Gently mash avocados in a medium-sized bowl, leaving some chunks. Add remaining ingredients and stir well to combine. If refrigerating, place pits on top of guacamole to prevent browning. Cover and chill.

Serve with sliced freshed veggies of your choice.

# SUNDAY

## Lunch:

### TERIYAKI TEMPEH WITH ASPARAGUS ARTICHOKE SALAD

- 1 8-ounce package tempeh, cut into 4 triangles
- ¼ cup Bragg's Liquid Aminos
- 1 tablespoon balsamic vinegar
- 3 tablespoons rice vinegar
- 4 drops pure stevia extract
- 1 inch piece fresh ginger, grated
- 3 cloves minced garlic
- 1 tablespoon sesame oil

Place tempeh in baking dish. Blend remaining ingredients. Pour over tempeh and refrigerate for 20 to 40 min. Preheat oven to 350°F. Cover tempeh with foil and bake for about 15 min, turning at least once. Uncover and cook for 5 more minutes.

### ASPARAGUS ARTICHOKE SALAD:

- 1 tablespoon olive oil
- ½ diced yellow onion
- 3 thinly sliced shiitake mushrooms
- 1 bunch asparagus, chopped
- 1 can artichoke hearts, drained, rinsed, and roughly chopped
- 4 sundried tomatoes, soaked and julienned
- 15 black olives, halved
- 1 teaspoon thyme
- 2 tablespoons balsamic vinegar
- 2 tablespoons water

Heat oil in skillet over medium heat and sauté onion and mushrooms. Add artichoke hearts, asparagus, tomatoes, olives, thyme, balsamic vinegar, and water. Cover and cook for about 5 to 7 minutes or until asparagus is tender and artichoke hearts are warmed through.

## Afternoon Snack:

**Hummus with fresh, raw veggies**

## MONDAY

Dinner:

**MISO STIR-FRY VEGGIES WITH TEMPEH OVER QUINOA OR BROWN RICE**

1 8-ounce package tempeh, cubed
1 tablespoon coconut oil
2 cloves minced garlic
1 teaspoon grated fresh ginger
1 thinly sliced small red onion
1 cup thinly sliced mushrooms
4 carrots, cut into ¼-inch rounds
1 zucchini, cut into ¼-inch rounds
1 cup broccoli florets
1 red bell pepper, julienned
1 cup chopped bok choy or cabbage

SAUCE:
2 cloves minced garlic
1 tablespoon freshly grated ginger
3 tablespoons mellow white miso
4 drops stevia extract
2 tablespoons low-sodium tamari
2 tablespoons toasted sesame oil
2 teaspoons arrowroot powder
Pinch red pepper flakes
½ cup coconut milk, full-fat, in can

Blend all sauce ingredients until smooth. In a large wok or sauté pan, heat oil over medium-high heat. Add garlic, onion, and ginger and sauté for 3 minutes or until onion is translucent. Add the remaining vegetables and stir to combine. Continue to sauté, about 5 minutes. Add the miso sauce and allow vegetables to cook in sauce for a few more minutes until sauce thickens. Remove from heat and serve over quinoa or brown rice.

## TUESDAY

Dinner:

**VEGGIE BURGERS AND QUINOA TABBOULEH**

1 15–ounce can chickpeas or 1½ cups cooked
1 cup cooked brown rice
½ red bell pepper, cut into chunks
½ onion, cut into chunks
1 cup baby spinach
Handful fresh cilantro
1½ cup gluten-free breadcrumbs
2 tablespoons tomato paste
½ teaspoon chili powder

Pulse chickpeas and brown rice together in food processor about 10 times. Scrape into large bowl. Puree bell pepper, onion, cilantro, and spinach in food processor until well combined; mixture will be very wet. Transfer mixture into bowl with the chickpea mixture. Stir in bread-crumbs, tomato paste, chili powder, salt, and pepper. Hand mix to combine ingredients. Form mixture into patties and heat on grill or skillet with olive oil until golden brown.

QUINOA TABBOULEH:
1 cup quinoa
2 cups water
½ cup chopped fresh mint
½ cup chopped fresh parsley
1 cup cucumber, peeled and diced
1 cup halved cherry tomatoes
2 tablespoons olive oil
2 cloves minced garlic
¼ cup lemon juice

Cook quinoa according to package directions. Once cooked, transfer to a large bowl to cool. Combine with remaining ingredients and stir to combine. Add sea salt and pepper to taste.

## WEDNESDAY

Dinner:

**WHITE BEAN AND SWEET POTATO SOUP WITH LARGE GREEN SALAD**

2 tablespoons olive oil
1 diced large yellow onion
3 cloves minced garlic
3 stalks diced celery
2 large sweet potatoes or garnet yams, peeled and cubed
2 cans white beans, drained and rinsed
1 teaspoon dried sage
1 teaspoon thyme
6 cups veggie broth or 3 bullion cubes with 6 cups water
2 tablespoons nutritional yeast

In a stock pot over medium heat, sauté onion, garlic, and celery in oil until soft. Add sage and thyme and stir to combine. Add sweet potatoes, white beans, and broth. Bring to a boil, turn heat to low, cover pot, and simmer until sweet potatoes are soft, about 20 to 30 minutes. Add sea salt to taste and stir in nutritional yeast.

# THURSDAY

## Dinner:

### SPAGHETTI SQUASH WITH MARINARA AND QUINOA TABBOULEH

1 cup quinoa
2 cups water
½ cup chopped fresh mint
½ cup chopped fresh parsley
1 cup diced cucumber, peeled
1 cup halved cherry tomatoes
2 tablespoons olive oil
2 cloves minced garlic
¼ cup lemon juice

Cook quinoa according to package directions. Once cooked, transfer to a large bowl to cool. Combine with all remaining ingredients and stir to combine. Season with sea salt and pepper to taste.

# FRIDAY

## Dinner:

### BLACK BEAN SWEET POTATO CHILI, BROWN RICE, AND SAUTÉED GARLIC BROCCOLI

2 tablespoons olive oil or coconut oil
1 chopped red bell pepper
1 medium diced red onion
4 cloves minced garlic
2 teaspoons sea salt
1 large garnet yam, peeled and cut into ½-inch cubes
Zest and juice of 1 lime
1 28-ounce can of fire-roasted, crushed tomatoes
3 cans black beans, drained & rinsed (or 4 cups freshly cooked)
1 tablespoon cumin
1 tablespoon chili powder
1 teaspoon cocoa powder
1 cup chopped cilantro for garnish (optional)

In large pot, heat oil over medium heat and sauté garlic, onion, red pepper, and sea salt until soft (about 4 to 5 min). Add the cumin and chili powder and stir to combine. Cook for another minute. Add chopped sweet potato and lime zest, cooking about 10 minutes more, stirring occasionally. Add the tomatoes, black beans, lime juice, and cocoa powder. Bring to a simmer, cover, and cook for about 10 minutes, or until potatoes are soft. Top with chopped cilantro.

# SATURDAY

## Dinner:

### TERIYAKI TEMPEH WITH QUINOA AND KALE SALAD WITH MISO DRESSING

1 8-ounce package tempeh, cut into 4 triangles
¼ cup Bragg's Liquid Aminos
1 tablespoon balsamic vinegar
3 tablespoons rice vinegar
4 drops pure stevia extract
1 inch piece fresh ginger, grated
3 cloves minced garlic
1 tablespoon sesame oil

Place tempeh in baking dish. Blend remaining ingredients together. Pour over tempeh and refrigerate for 20 to 40 min. Preheat oven to 350°F. Cover tempeh with foil and bake for about 15 min, turning at least once. Uncover and cook for 5 more minutes.

KALE SALAD WITH MISO DRESSING:
1 head kale, destemmed and chopped
1 tablespoon olive oil
¼ cup pine nuts
½ cup halved cherry tomatoes
¼ cup thinly sliced fennel
Miso dressing (See recipe below.)

Place kale in a large salad bowl and drizzle with olive oil and dash of salt. Massage kale for a few minutes until it softens. This makes the kale more digestable. Add tomatoes, fennel, and pine nuts. Toss with miso dressing.

MISO DRESSING:
1 diced shallot
1 tablespoon Dijon mustard
1 tablespoon mellow white miso
¼ cup unsweetened, rice vinegar
4 drops stevia extract
3 tablespoons olive oil

Blend in a blender cup or shake well to mix.

# SUNDAY

## Dinner:

### COCONUT YAM SOUP

2 Garnet yams, peeled and cubed
3 large carrots, peeled and diced
2 celery stalks, diced
1 large yellow onion, diced
1 leek, thinly sliced
3 cloves minced garlic
1 teaspoon fresh ginger, optional
2 teaspoon Garam Masala (indian spice)
4 cups veggie broth
1 tablespoon coconut or olive oil
1 can coconut milk
Sea salt and fresh cracked pepper
Cinnamon and nutmeg for garnish

In a large soup pot over medium heat, saute ginger, garlic, celery, onion and leek in oil until translucent and soft. Add Garam Masala and stir to combine to release the flavor of the spice. Add the carrots, yams, and veggie broth. Turn heat to high and bring to a boil. Once it reaches boiling, cover and turn heat down to a simmer. Let simmer for 20-30 minutes, or until veggies are tender. Remove from heat and add coconut milk. Puree soup using a hand blender until thick and creamy. Season with salt and pepper and garnish with a dash of cinnamon and nutmeg!

Variation: Add 1 cup of red lentils to soup while cooking and increase water by 1 cup.

# ACKNOWLEDGMENTS

C reating this book has been a journey, with a number of Sherpas who helped chart the path. Leading the way were my editors, Krista Lyons and Merrik Bush, and the team at Seal Press who helped bring my vision to life: publicist Eva Zimmerman, and book designers Megan Jones and Tabitha Lahr. A big sun salutation to Erika Lenkert, who guided me and gave me the confidence to feel I could actually write a book and who helped nurture me every step of the way. Thanks also to Shab Azma and Robert Flutie for connecting me with my agents, Jane Dystel and Miriam Goderich, who educated me through the process, listened to my opinions, and have been as steadfast and grounding as tree pose.

Thanks, as always, for the assist from Jenni Anspach, who helps keep an eye on the group with her tireless service. I would be remiss if I did not acknowledge my awesome education in the school of experiential learning: Life. A big, strong warrior pose is in order for teachers Craig McEwen, Sally Lew, Fred Donaldson, and Rolf McEwen, who gave me permission to whack the bell curve right in half and to unlearn, question authority, and explore the big wide word through MOBOC (Mobile Open Classrooms).

Big props also to my acting teachers, especially Diane Hardin, who encouraged me to go big and follow my dreams with the magic words "I believe in you." Likewise to the myriad of teachers, acting and fitness alike, Joanne Baron, and Julie Ariola, who trained me to be a shamanic artist; and my original yoga teacher, Lloyd Ingber.

Other notables: Baron Baptiste, Candace Copeland, Johnny G, Bob Harper, Bryan Kest, Keshava Kronish, and Billy Porter; and the many authors and artists, philosophers, and actors who have informed and inspired me. To my dear friends, who teach me to look within and fill my own cup first. You know who you are.

To my talented, beautification team, photographer Javiera Estrada, makeup artist Glen Alen, and wardrobe gal Jill McDonald. To Jeff Christensen and his staff at Kinevision Studio in Venice, California. To my loyal clients, notably Jennifer Aniston, who pointed the finger my direction; and especially to my greatest teachers, the many students that I have been blessed with teaching since 1996: Thank you for teaching me that loving is above giving.

To my younger siblings—Dave, Max, and Megan—who teach me that being older doesn't mean knowing more. To my favorite grandmother, Bubbie Sonia, who taught me that being older is an illusion anyway. To my first teacher, my mom, Linda Ingber, a teacher still. Thank you, Mom, for teaching me how to read, write, draw, speak, identify a parallelogram and a trapezoid, and the names of the dinosaurs and the Greek Gods. And for turning me on to Steve Martin. Thank you for being curious. And for always staying childlike. Lastly, I want to tip my hat to the great teacher: God. Life. Universal Love. The Divine Mother. Grace. Whatever you want to call it. Thank you for always directing me from within to the next right action.

# ABOUT THE AUTHOR

Mandy Ingber is a Los Angeles-based fitness and wellness expert whose sold-out classes have set the precedent for more than twenty years. Following a successful career as a young actress—during which she originated the role of "Laurie" in Neil Simon's acclaimed stage play *Brighton Beach Memoirs*; had memorable parts on such hit television shows as *Cheers, Charles in Charge,* and *My Sister Sam*; and costarred in the beloved contemporary classic film *Teen Witch*—she transitioned into the world of fitness.

Ingber's notable roster of clients includes Jennifer Aniston, Kate Beckinsale, Academy Award-winner Helen Hunt (who credits Mandy with getting her body "Oscar-ready" for the red carpet), Brooke Shields, and jewelry designer Jennifer Meyer Maguire. She blogs regularly about health and wellness for E! online and People.com and has been named the "Best of LA" in *LA Weekly* and *Los Angeles* magazines for her motivation, inspiration, and the popularity of her classes. Her online contributions have ranged from Huffington Post to Yahoo! Shine to Oprah.com. She is frequently featured on network television shows such as *Extra, The Today Show, Good Morning America Health, Access Hollywood, E! Entertainment,* and *Good Day LA,* as well as in magazines such as *Self, InStyle, Elle, USWeekly, People, Vogue, Women's Health, O, Shape, Glamour, Good Housekeeping,* and *Los Angeles.*

For more information, visit mandyingber.com.

# INDEX

# SELECTED TITLES FROM SEAL PRESS

*BEAUTIFUL YOU: A DAILY GUIDE TO RADICAL SELF-ACCEPTANCE*, by Rosie Molinary. $16.95, 978-1-58005-331-0. A practical, accessible, day-by-day guide to redefining beauty and building lasting self-esteem from body expert Rosie Molinary.

*AIRBRUSHED NATION: THE LURE AND LOATHING OF WOMEN'S MAGAZINES*, by Jennifer Nelson. $17.00, 978-1-58005-413-3. Jennifer Nelson—a longtime industry insider—exposes the naked truth behind the glossy pages of women's magazines, both good and bad.

*DANCING AT THE SHAME PROM: SHARING THE STORIES THAT KEPT US SMALL*, edited by Amy Ferris and Hollye Dexter. $15.00, 978-1-58005-416-4. A collection of funny, sad, poignant, miraculous, life-changing, and jaw-dropping secrets for readers to gawk at, empathize with, and laugh about—in the hopes that they will be inspired to share their secret burdens as well.

*1,000 MITZVAHS: HOW SMALL ACTS OF KINDNESS CAN HEAL, INSPIRE, AND CHANGE YOUR LIFE*, by Linda Cohen. $16.00, 978-1-58005-365-5. When her father passes away, Linda Cohen decides to perform one thousand mitzvahs, or acts of kindness, to honor his memory—and discovers the transformational power of doing good for others.

*ABOUT FACE: WOMEN WRITE ABOUT WHAT THEY SEE WHEN THEY LOOK IN THE MIRROR*, edited by Anne Burt and Christina Baker Kline. $15.95, 978-1-58005-246-7. Twenty-five women writers candidly examine their own faces—and each face has a story to tell.

*RUN LIKE A GIRL: HOW STRONG WOMEN MAKE HAPPY LIVES*, by Mina Samuels. $16.95, 978-1-58005-345-7. Author and athlete Mina Samuels writes about how lessons learned on the field (or track, or slopes) can help us face challenges in other areas—and how, for many women, participating in sports translates into leading a happier, more fulfilling life.

FIND SEAL PRESS ONLINE

www.SealPress.com

www.Facebook.com/SealPress

Twitter: @SealPress